# Heal Psoriasis at the Dead Sea

## Matthew Allen

Copyright 2018 by Matthew Allen
All rights reserved.
Smashwords Edition

HealthRightISRAEL
Monsey, New York
www.HealthRightIsrael.com

Smashwords Edition, License Notes



**CONTENTS**

## INTRODUCTION

This book is a personal story of recovery and managing chronic psoriasis for over 25 years of my life. It was written in three stages 2007, 2013 and finally 2017, spanning ten years of travel to Israel, researching this project plus two and a half years of living in Israel…experiencing firsthand the healing powers of the Dead Sea. I have come to believe this ancient basin of hot mineral waters in Israel, deep below sea level, is one of the most mysterious and healing spots on Earth.

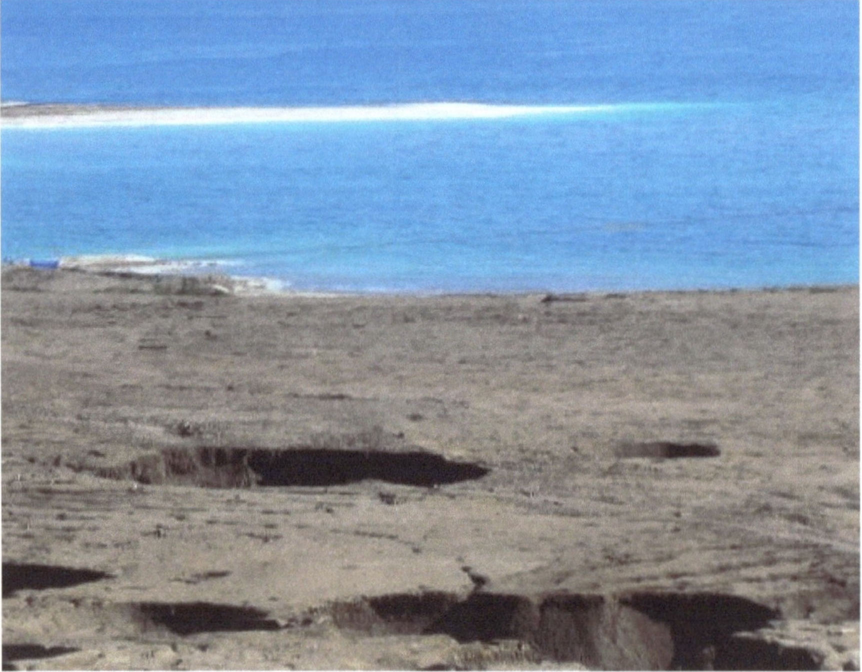

It's a saga of rejuvenation and rejoicing following over ten years of individualized experimentation with psoriasis treatment in a clinical spa at the lowest point on the Earth, the basin Israeli people often call the "Great Salty Sea." In Hebrew it translates to *Yam Hamelach*. While it appears to be a rather lifeless desert region, the Dead Sea is very alive.

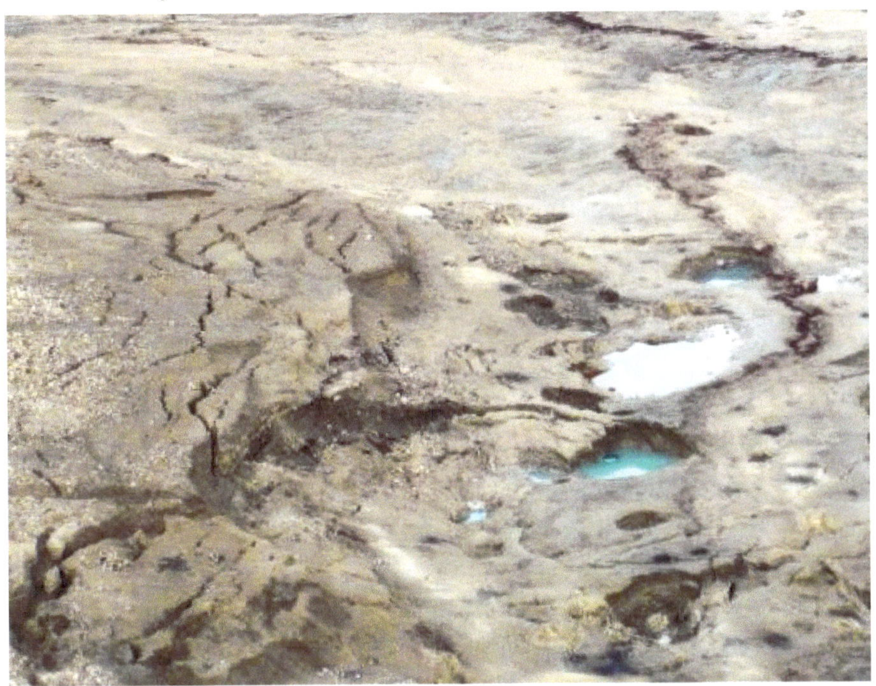

## HISTORICAL BACKGROUND ON THE REGION

A little historical orientation of the area is required. Below on the left image is an aerial shot taken in 1970 showing how much water was present compared to a more recent photo in 2013. A dam was placed above the Jordan River, the tributary to this historical wonder. Its purpose was for agricultural irrigation by Israel and Jordan, however, it has created a great controversy in both countries since Israel became a world leader in water desalination. There actually is no further need to dam the Jordan River above the Dead Sea for fresh water. Israel can irrigate at will from any water source. The other major reason for concern and controversy is that the Dead Sea waters have been receding so much that land is caving in around the Dead Sea causing sinkholes which damage local nature sites, animal life and the nearby hotel/spa industries.

The major change from this initial photo on the left to the one on its right (taken 33 years later) demonstrates the disappearance of part of the lower sea region—stemming from a significant decline in the amount of water reaching it via tributaries, as mentioned.

The sea level is dropping by about one meter per year, exposing large areas of soft earth to deep and dangerous hidden caverns called sinkholes. In 1970, the level of the Dead Sea was measured at 395 meters below sea level. By 2013 this level sunk another 32 meters to an astonishing 427 meters below sea level (which is a dangerous drop of 197 feet in water levels since 1970).

Some of the surrounding landscape was affected by digging and quarrying by the Dead Sea Works Company for salts and minerals. In addition, major cosmetics are mined and sold by regional companies.

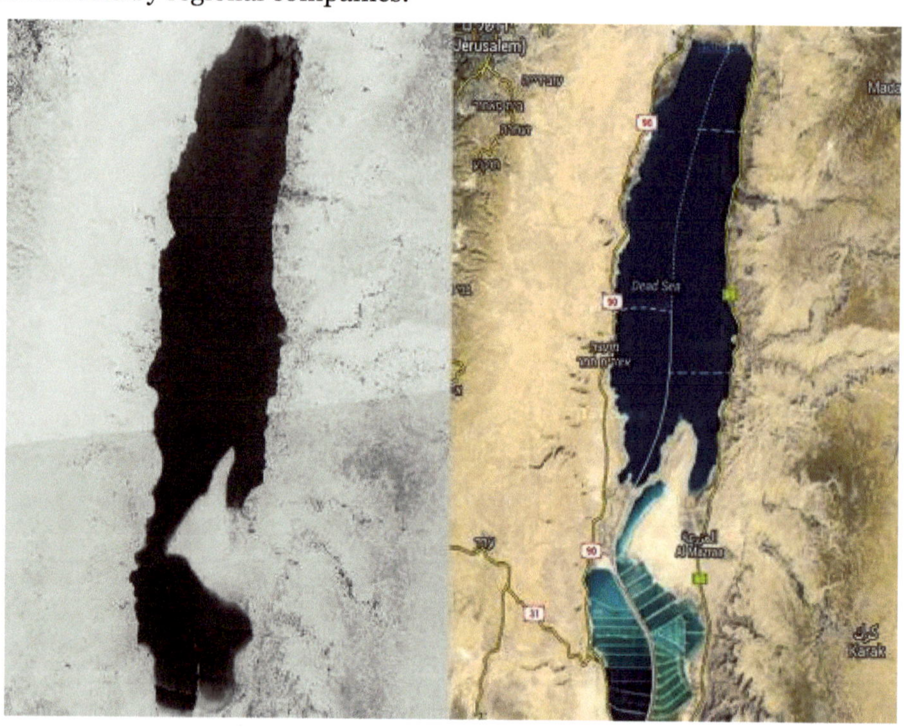


(Source www.haaretz.com)

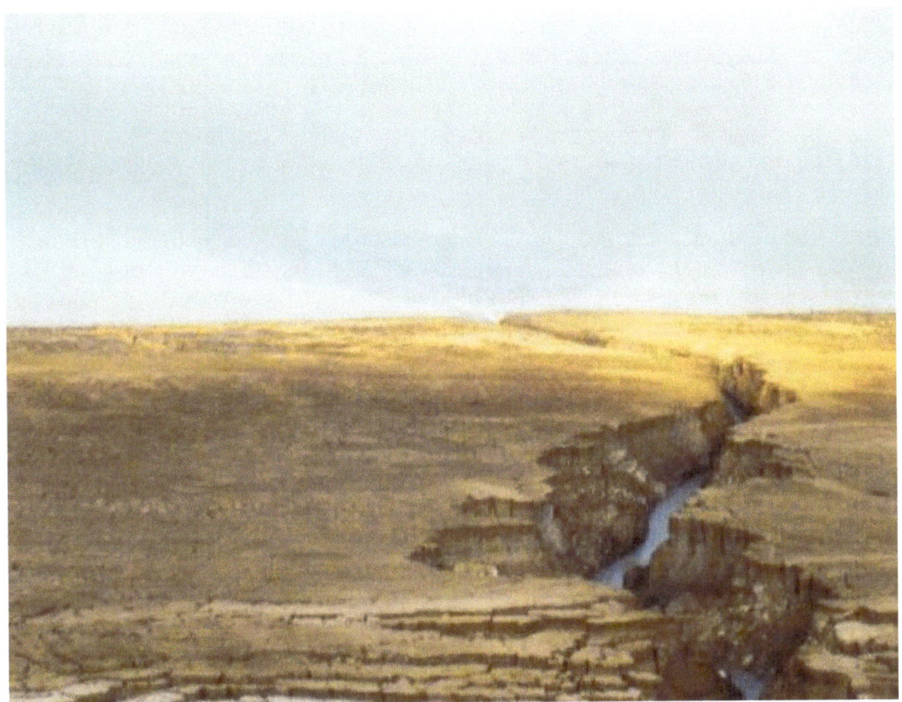

Many people think of the Dead Sea as being lifeless, and how could life exist in this hot, dense, mineral body of water whose average temperature is a scorching 75-90 degrees Fahrenheit?

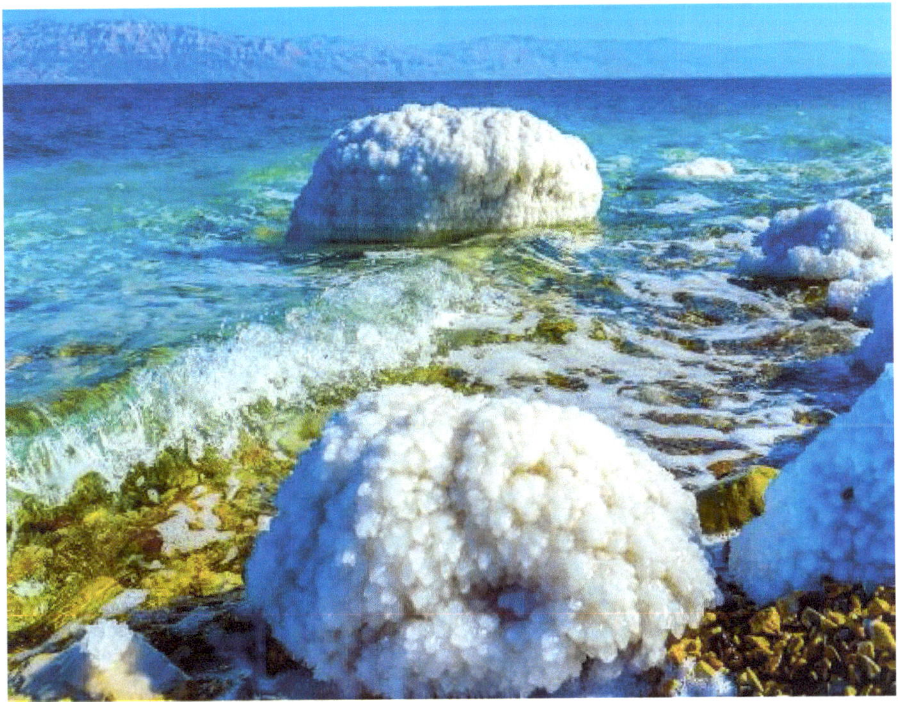

In reality, both microbial creatures and even small fish have been discovered by scientists deep in its undercurrent streams. Also, consider the constantly growing salt mineral crystals everywhere in and out of the water. Do they grow and live?

This is a real myth-buster since so many people say there can be no life at the Dead Sea. But, for people who have stayed there more than a day or two, we all know the Dead Sea is "beaming with vitality!"

Perhaps, original map makers took their cue from stories told by early Roman conquerors of the Holy Land. We know that Caesar himself left his mark on the shores of Israel because we find ancient aqueduct and Colosseum ruins of his culture in the city of Caesarea on the Israeli Mediterranean Sea. Ironically, in writing this journal, I saw ruins of Caesarea while on a train making all coastal stops from Haifa to Tel Aviv. Caesar's loyal subject, King Herod had his architects build these amazing structures. Herod also erected the magnificent fortress known as Masada, which was one of Herod's royal palaces high on a mountaintop overlooking the Dead Sea. Here a band of Jewish zealots perished because they resisted conquest by these Roman Legions. The Romans had already destroyed Jerusalem killing thousands and these were the last rebels remaining. Masada is an amazing story of holding out for life under unbearable circumstances. In our history, Jewish stories tell us that rather than giving up to the Romans, the Jews committed mass suicide.

During the same period of this conquest, stories have been passed down that one of Caesar's soldiers may have drunk from these poisoned mineral waters and died shortly after. Perhaps this is why it's now called the Dead Sea.

Thousands of years ago Cleopatra laid claim to the curative powers of this amazing water and its soothing minerals as promoting great health and longevity to those who happened upon it, bathed and took in the glorious sun rays.

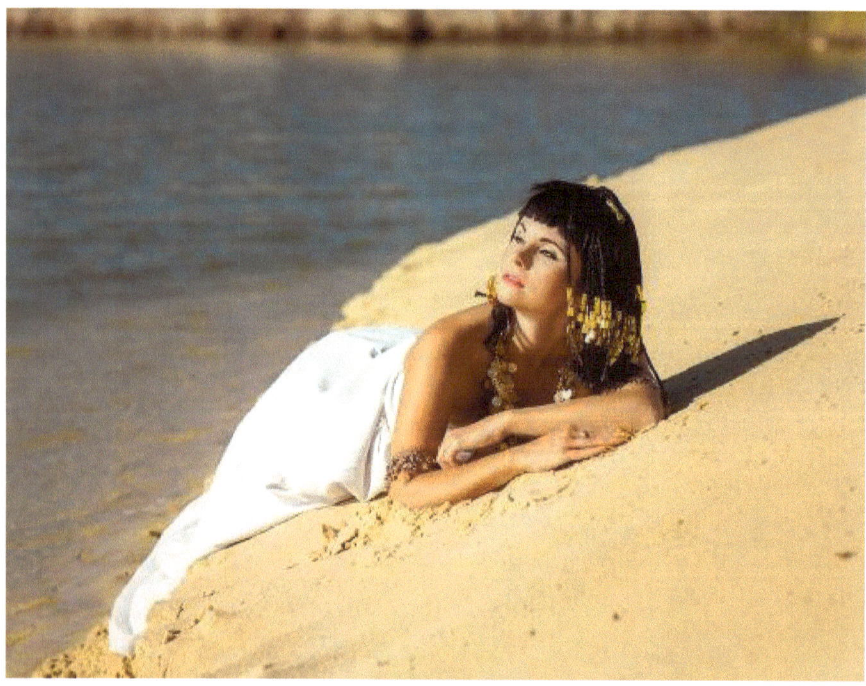

© *Elena Brodetskaya / Adobe Stock*

Today, and for more than 60 years, many Westerners and Europeans have traveled at great expense to Dead Sea hotels and clinics to heal with these salty and mineral-rich waters plus its unique safe UVB rays of sunlight. In the last ten years, I stayed there multiple times for entire summers. And, I have experienced that the Dead Sea is very much alive. It breathes and brings forth revitalization to all who come and bathe in its amazing waters while tanning in those special sunrays. While a short vacation at the Dead Sea is wonderful...for skin, joint, and other acute treatments a three to four-week stay is necessary.

**Now that you see the Dead Sea is alive, here's my personal story**

As a victim of psoriasis, I've had major relief and recovery after repeatedly going to this special place—having had chronic psoriasis on 80% of my skin from head-to-toe for over 25 years. Sometimes it's better, sometimes worse, but on the shores of the Dead Sea, Israel's eighth wonder of the world, my red and flaky skin "magically" melts away!

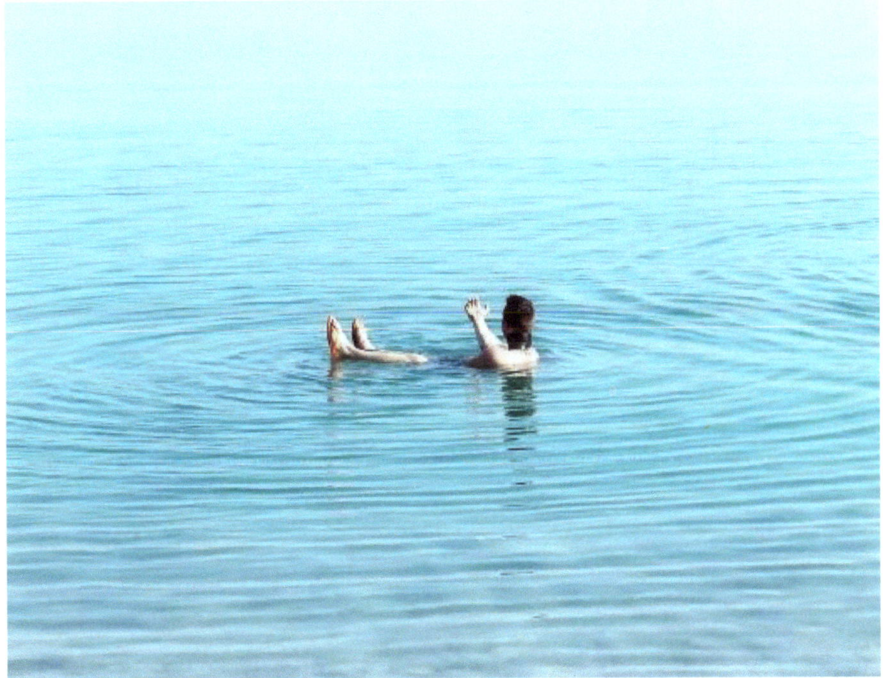

By some miracle, this natural deep mineral sea with its unique sunrays has repeatedly cleared my skin in 14-21 days, like clockwork. In this book you will learn how.

## DIMONA'S BLACK HEBREW NUTRITION PROGRAM

During my 2017 extended stay in Israel, I met the Black Hebrew tribal elders of Dimona who call the Dead Sea the "Sea of Life" due to its vast curative minerals plus rejuvenation history. In this fourth cleansing visit, I made a major shift in my food intake while repeating the sea and sun treatment as before. I decided to eat mostly vegan meals with the exception of eggs and herring in olive oil for breakfast. For the rest of my lunches and dinners during the four weeks at the Dead Sea, I ate only fresh live or cooked foods prepared by these Black Hebrews north of the Dead Sea region in a city called Dimona.

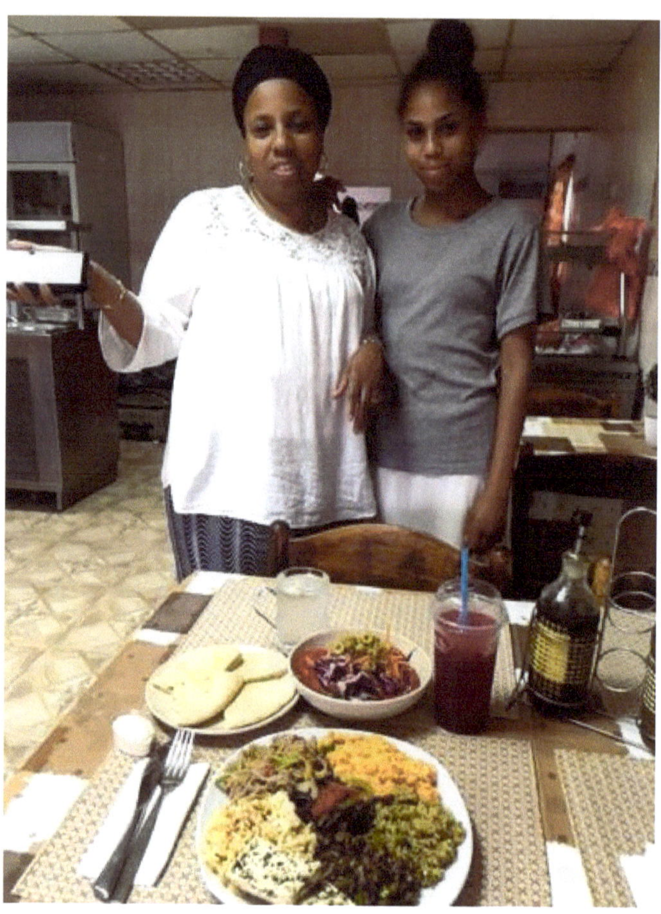

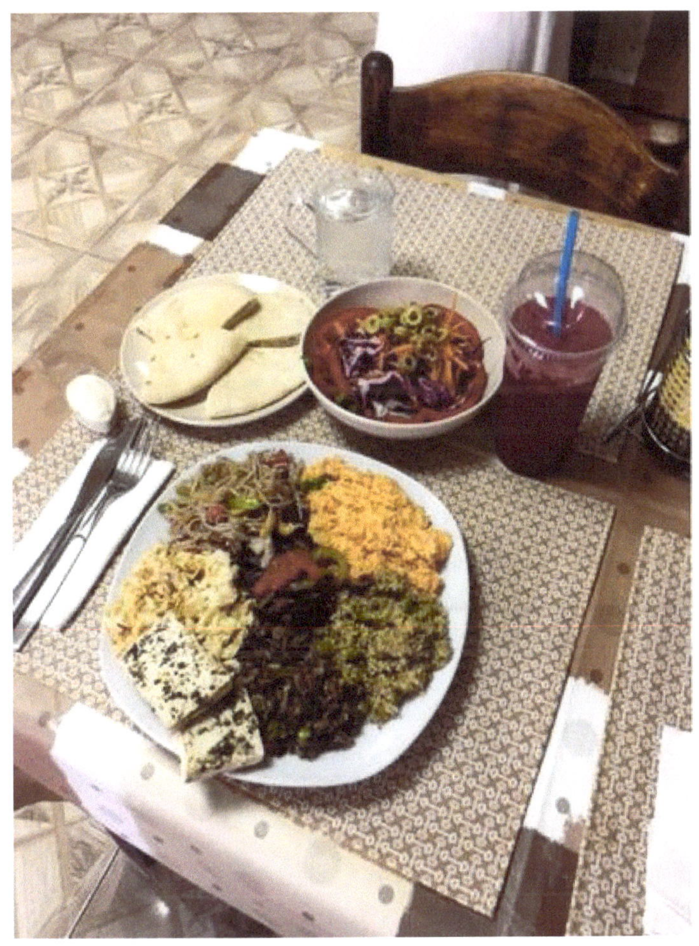

Historically, this small group of 3,000 Black Hebrews settled in Israel (leaving Chicago, Detroit and other places of segregation and brutality) during the 1960s when civil rights horrors were occurring in America. They chose this place to raise future generations in joy, health and peace, close to the origin of all nations—Mesopotamia—where they believe our common ancestors came from.

Rightfully, they have called it the Village of Peace where I went every Sunday, Tuesday and Thursday to learn about their culture and enjoy the bountiful food in their vegan restaurant, open to the public.

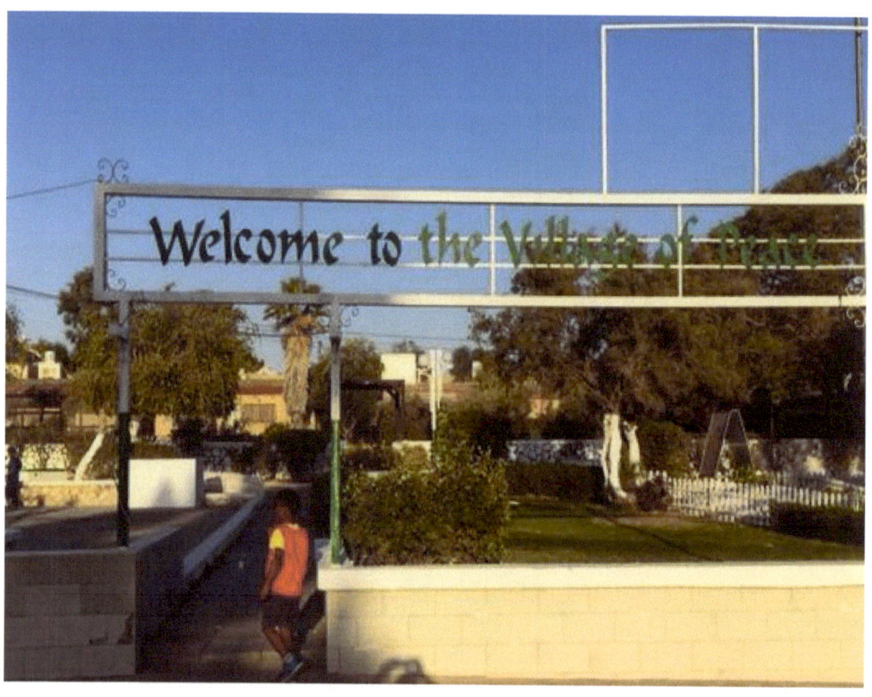


Together with the guidance of their elders and nutrition healers, I have created this chapter to encourage visitors to the Dead Sea region to include this menu while they heal from autoimmune conditions like psoriasis and arthritis.

The food was delicious and bountiful. Every day I arrived, the plate they served me was enough for three meals. So, I just took a doggy bag and ate it for lunch and dinner the next few days. They taught me that all wellness requires lifestyle commitments and they have witnessed great health and longevity when their villagers observe five basic rules: mandatory exercise, vegan food, periodic fasting, mindfulness, proper rest and relaxation, attention to digestion and elimination. All of this is posted on a sign in their gymnasium.

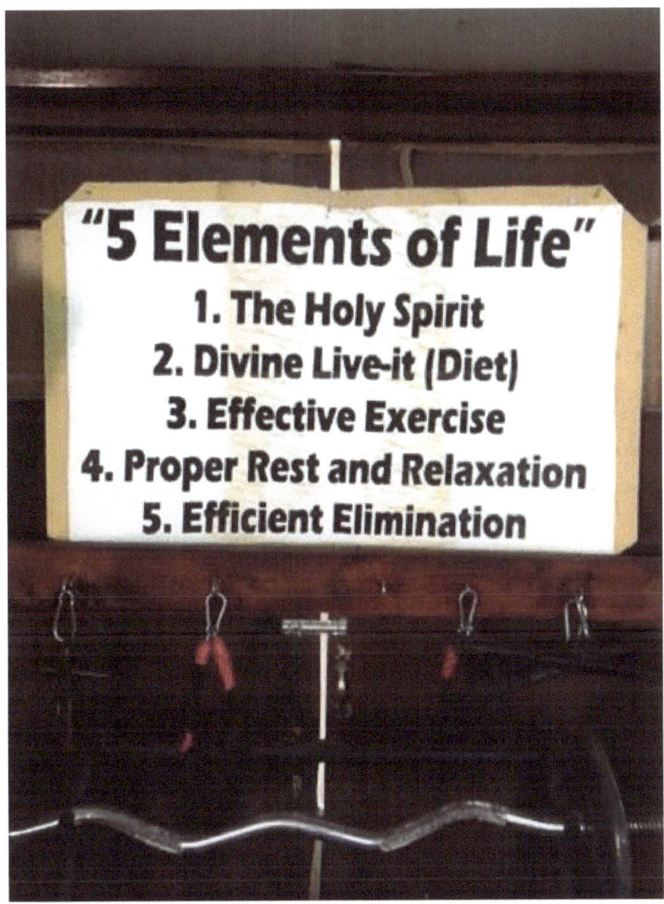



This Village of Peace ambassador Yoyah, below, a second-generation man in his mid-twenties told me what I had already seen in a graphical movie about racial hatred and atrocities in Chicago, Detroit, New York, L.A. and most of the southern USA during the early 1960s. This killing trend continued up to and beyond the assassinations of Malcolm X, Dr. Martin Luther King, Jr., and both Kennedy's. It goes on now with terrorism and mass murders globally. All of this bigotry and murder led a group of about 500 Blacks to make their "first Exodus," as he described it, to Liberia, for a period lasting three to four years. Many struggled and 75% returned to the USA due to hardships and lack of true grit commitment.

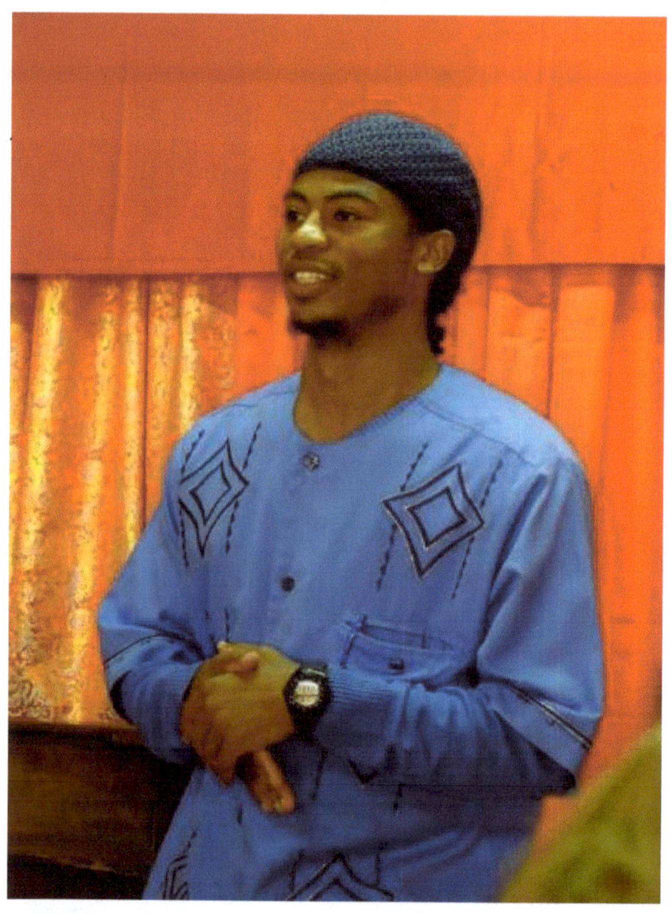

Of those who survived, they made a "second Exodus" to Israel's Holy Promised Land. Israel approved their immigration as a lost Hebrew non-Jewish tribe from Africa. While believing in one G-d they don't practice religious traditions except for blessings on their vegan food. They also celebrate every Sabbath by fasting all day. They explained this practice to me in two ways. First, if G-d rested on the seventh day of creation, then why don't we practice doing nothing as well on that day? Secondly, fasting is both a spiritual cleansing and detox method for healing which goes back beyond Moses.

I learned more details from my next interview with Almadiel Ben Yehuda, (next to me below, on my left) Minister of Information and National Spokesman who arrived in the 1970s as a youth in his 20s. From a mere 500 villagers who immigrated in 1969, they currently have grown to over 3,000 in the community just 48 years later. Part of this amazing growth is due to their adopting the ancient African and Hebrew practice of multiple wives (polygany), resulting in multiple offspring, a common lifestyle which both Abraham and Jacob had in the Bible.

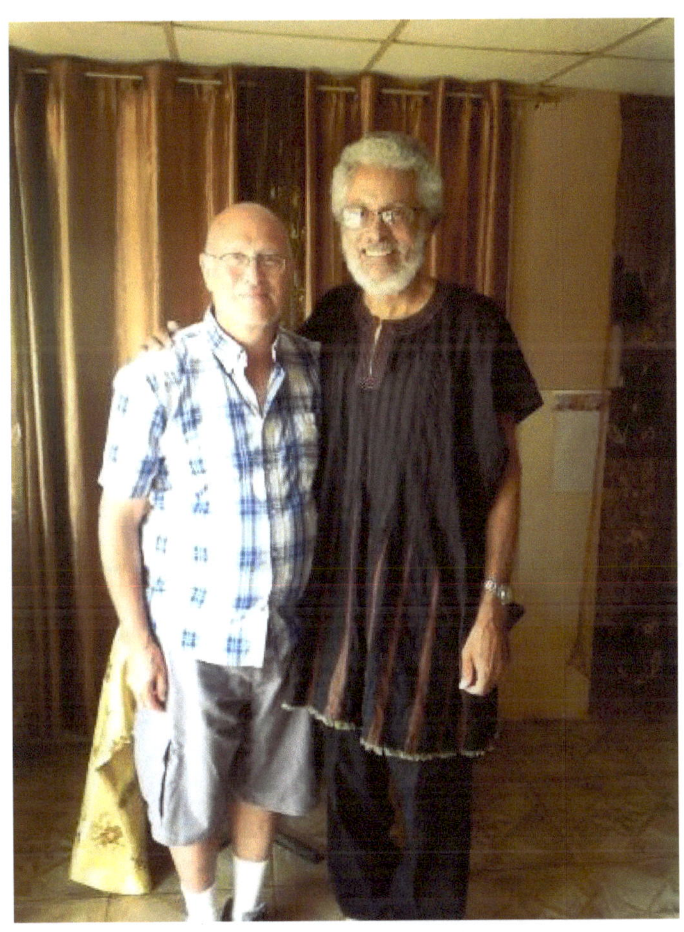

I then met with their medicine man, female nutritionist and the community ambassador, a very charismatic woman named Ahamalyah (on the right). The story of wonderful and joyous Ahamalyah's journey originated in Los Angeles, where she was an activist student. There she met and studied with the civil rights radical Stokely Carmichael, famous for his "Pan-African" work after his previous civil rights connections with Dr. Martin Luther King, Jr.

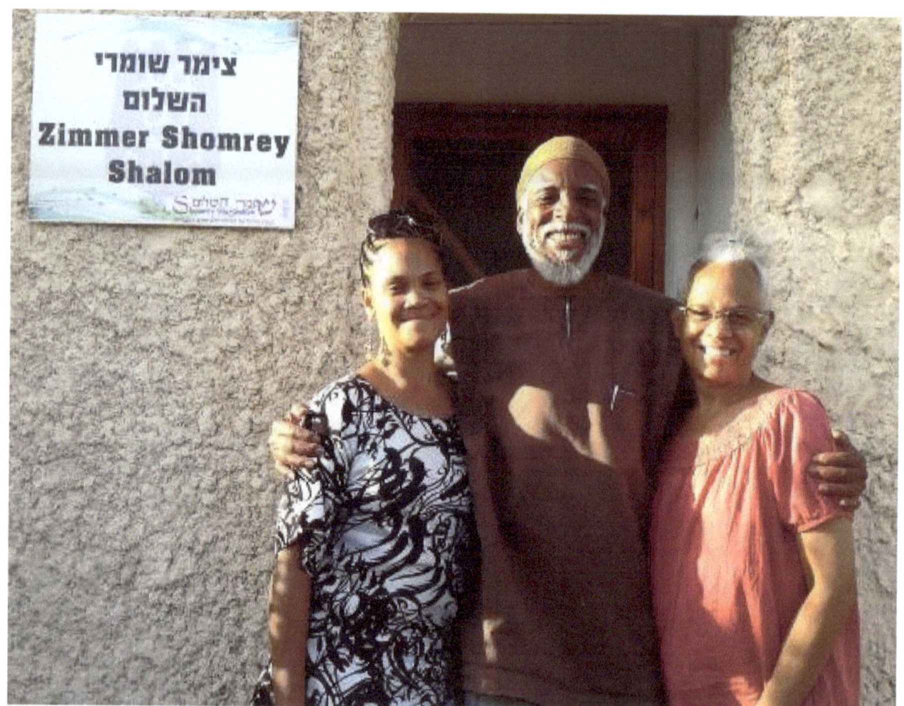


While at U.C. San Diego, Ahamalyah maintained a connection for seven years with Stokely's worldwide movement, whose mission was to strengthen relations with Africans everywhere. After this, in 1984 she decided to sojourn across the Atlantic directly to the city of Dimona, Israel with her husband from Chicago. She landed nine-months pregnant and gave birth to her son Zion (below).

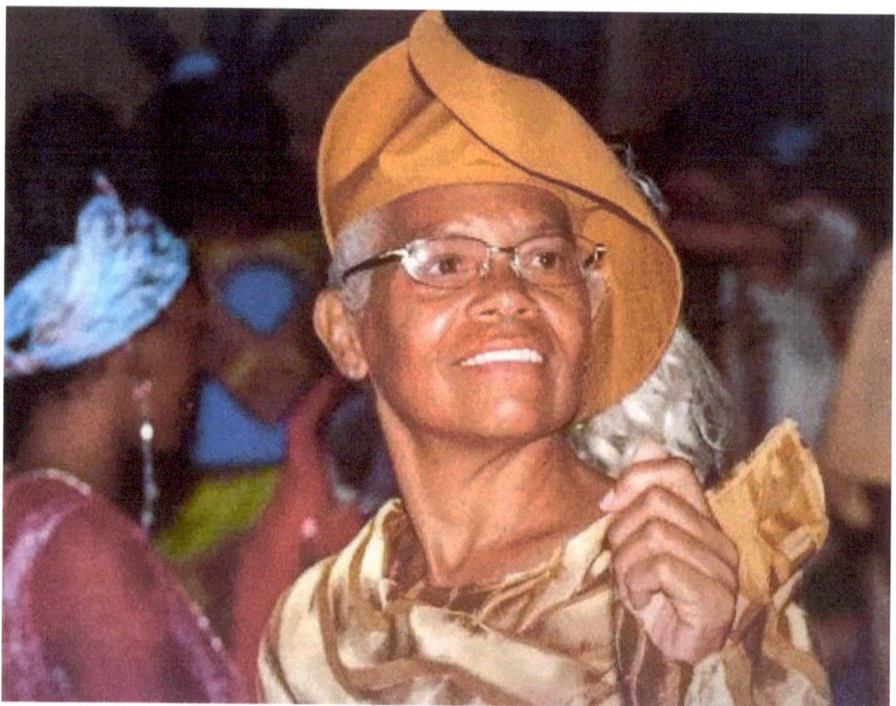

At the time of this photo he was 33, a proud father, and husband of a second-generation of returning Black Hebrews at the Village of Peace.

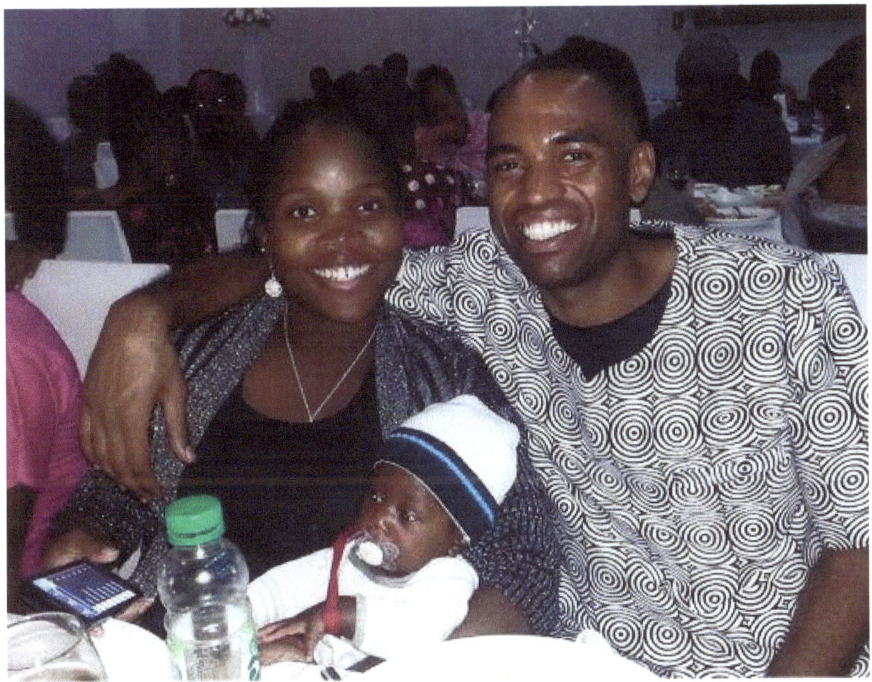

What is this Village of Peace about? What brought hundreds of Black Hebrews during decades of civil rights strife to Liberia first...then to Israel for asylum and peace, health and safety?

They came because of brutality in the US, but they discovered their own humanity by thoroughly researching their Hebrew past and their inheritance. This knowledge gave them a purpose and a mission, leading to their naming their place "Village of Peace." In talking with the elders about this name, they agreed it should include the ideas of health, harmony and community. Therefore, the word peace may confuse outsiders which is why people need to experience and appreciate where the Black Hebrews are coming from.

Since a health and wellness lifestyle is the significant part of this journal, I have found that nutrition is an essential aspect of inside healing...directly affecting digestion, elimination and our skin reactions.

At the Village of Peace, using vegan recipes developed in the 1960s, a grandmother, her daughter and grandson created many recipes derived from ancient texts such as the Bible and were intended to be similar to those foods consumed by our ancestors in the region. Her grandson Yihoyakeem (seen below at their new restaurant) and his mother Yesha, a nutritionist, are writing a four-generations vegan cookbook in honor of his grandmother who recently passed away. I'm told grandma was a wonderful woman and an amazing chef. Indeed, her nutritionist daughter along with her son Yihoyakeem are dedicated to keeping the vegan food preparation alive for the next generations at the Village of Peace. I also visited Yihoyakeem in Tel Aviv at their recent opening of *The Taste of Life* vegan deli, where they offer this cuisine in a more metropolitan market of Israel.

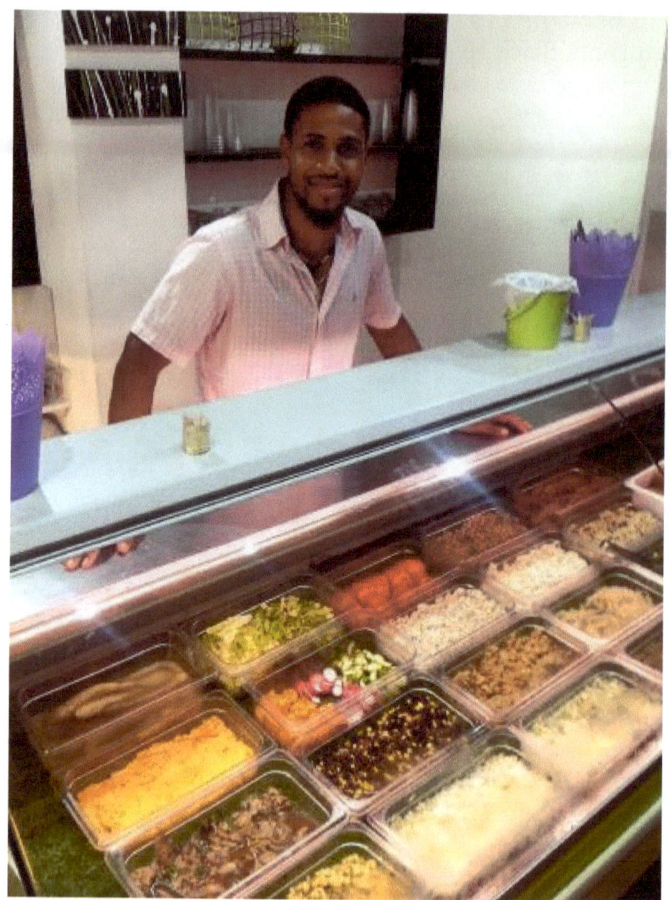

The villagers are to be admired and learned from—their adherence to the *5 Elements of Life* has led to their joy and longevity. It's a potential story of how we may all find a way to return to youthful wellness before the stresses of life took over. Here is a useful link to raw vegan recipes at www.rawfoodforlife.org which may be helpful in your quest for better health.



### My health journey begins here

It's not every day you can confront and conquer a condition as annoying as the "heartbreak of psoriasis." At age 28, my skin first erupted, displaying itchy redness on 80% of my body.

Through the years, I realized it was really a battle with my own recurring inner monsters. Two ugly themes surfaced, one of personal shame in looking so red and spotted in public, and the other theme was just not knowing how to let go of the depression surrounding long-lasting, acute psoriasis.

Rooted in a dysfunctional childhood, no one ever guided this adorable young Matthew out of his childhood shame and related fears. As you can see, I started out as a very healthy, beautiful and innocent boy. I so remember this beautiful inner child.

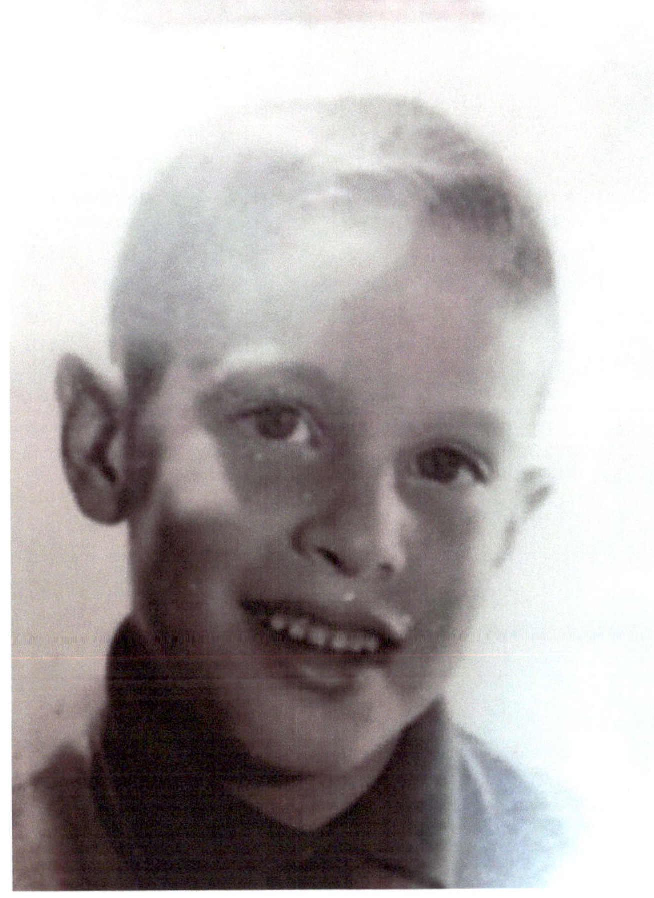

Up front, I want to share with you my sincere belief that what triggered my skin condition could have been avoided. It was connected to this early deep shame, which I feel led to my depression and compromised my internal organs. Furthermore, all of this intense emotion could have psychosomatically released dangerous toxins in my gut causing skin stress.

In alternative medicine, it is believed that psoriasis can be reversed with both nutrition and mindful attitude changes, yet allopathic Western medicine often holds that there is no cure.

It's always been up to me to accomplish changes in my health. Often taking this kind of responsibility is daunting. But it is possible. It's an individual journey beginning when we decide we no longer want to continue down an unhealthy path. We have to believe in our guts it can happen. And our gut plays a major part as we will discuss.

## My life's key events unfold

At 16, I had a very bad case of mononucleosis which put me in bed taking massive doses of antibiotics for about six months. Shortly after this, I had strep throat and due to this virus, doctors advised that I have my tonsils removed at age 19. I recall this was an excruciating operation. I can't express how much my throat burned for over two weeks. Many researchers have seen strep as a consistent trigger ailment to psoriasis at www.psoriasis.org/about-psoriasis/types/guttate. Soon I became aware of my weaker immune system functions. As I got older, I had Chronic Fatigue Syndrome for many years and became weak, lethargic and gained weight easily.

As I started to recover, slowly, I began to go to art school in New York City. At the School of Visual Art's I met and fell I head over heels for a beautiful French-speaking Haitian woman. Her line drawing was captivating, and this romantic encounter appeared as my first real love. We dated and I soon met her father, who was a master Haitian craftsman. He was an extraordinarily bold and precise painter, sculptor and Renaissance man. He could do anything in the visual arts. So, when by age 19, I witnessed two amazing artists, my own value and confidence dropped even more. While it I may have loved her, I was so confused, it seemed I adored what she and her father could do that I was unable able to. This envy increasingly diminished my sense of self-confidence and worth, clearly a factor in increasing shame. I thought, *What was wrong with me? Wasn't I a good enough artist.*

That summer, working as a sales clerk, I earned enough money to travel, (but it was actually to escape) to Europe where I enrolled in an arts and language program in Italy. I desperately needed to get away from my lack of confidence—a change of scenery, I imagined—would do me good. How wrong I would be!

It soon became clear you cannot run away from yourself. My journey to Italy became a fantasy into the world of amazing artists of the Renaissance such as Michelangelo, Leonardo da Vinci and countless others. It was a very self-destructive period of my youth where I became exceedingly euphoric—delusional in the midst of all of this amazing Italian beauty, color, art and grandeur.

Sexually, I also became very active, meeting beautiful Italian women in the piazzas and at nightclubs...subsequently having multiple relationships, running around town, into the hills and making myself into a braggart, nuisance and a spectacle.

My loving father was notified by my friend, an Italian teacher, to come and return me to the USA before anything worse could occur. My dad arrived, and with strong prescription medication he was able to subdue me and return me home, docile. I was soon hospitalized in the USA for two to three months, under observation and care for what appeared to be a mental breakdown.

The doctors later categorized this episode as a bipolar disorder. Whether properly diagnosed or not it required a medication. A strong side-effect of this drug became a rash of full body psoriasis skin eruptions. The drug, known as lithium carbonate, helped control my euphoria and kept me functioning at a very high level. I seemed fine during these years from 20 - 27, but by the age of 28, psoriasis was my new "best friend!" I've had it to some degree ever since.

After this brief hospitalization and my speedy recovery, I returned to my parent's home and commuted to city college. In three short years, I graduated with a B.A. major in anthropology and minor in studio art, both with high honors from Hunter College in New York City. Within three years, I went to graduate school in Albuquerque, New Mexico and enrolled in a master's program in computer science. In two more years, I became a "pseudo-geek" but decided to go into computer sales instead of programming. My eyesight was failing and I couldn't handle programming all day. One could say I couldn't "hack" it...ha, ha!

While living and working in NYC at around 27, I met my future wife to be at a Chinese New Year's party on lower Broadway in a loft. I noticed her beautiful curly blond hair and deep blue eyes immediately. Ironically, my Ronni and I dated only briefly before I went west to work in Hollywood's film business.

My wife and I soon rekindled our relationship long-distance and she later visited me one Thanksgiving at the computer graduate school in New Mexico, where we solidified our love and started a formal courtship. Within a year we were married and one year later had our first daughter, Alexandra.

To know what happened in these first 28 years of my life, before the blemishes of psoriasis emerged, you'd almost have to be a detective like Sherlock Holmes to uncover each clue of this gradual change in my health. It was not perceivable from my youth that this could possibly happen to me as, in my 25 years or more, I was extremely vigorous and courageous. Something unpredictable began to go wrong around the time I was married. I believe it was triggered around knowing how much I personally felt responsible and worried about providing for my family.

My brain seemed to be functioning well at the time, as I worked full-time in New York in computer marketing. However, I noticed my skin erupting with psoriasis around this time and my joints began swelling with arthritis. One of the first issues I noticed during this change in my health was also a chronic fatigue that made me very tired during the day and up late during the night.

I began to feel very mercurial. This was a symptom which soon showed me that I was toxic. I found out later, after doing a special hair analysis test, that my childhood dentist used a lot of mercury amalgam fillings in my teeth from age 10 - 18 which had subsequently leached into my blood, tissues and brain functions. I was clinically diagnosed with mercury poisoning. Mercury and lithium carbonate are both listed in the *Physicians' Desk Reference* book, as directly causing psoriasis. But, mercury also affects depression, chronic fatigue, and can cause bipolar mercurial behaviors. It appeared as though a string of health issues (mono, strep, tonsillectomy, excess mercury compounded with lithium treatment) may have indirectly caused my psoriasis with a weakening of my autoimmune system.

I increasingly broke out with red and scaly skin everywhere, and worse than all of this, I started to feel that the mercury itself may have caused my bipolar condition. To this day, no one can be certain.

My mention of mercury is critical since the use of mercury amalgam fillings in teeth has been used extensively in the Western world. The danger of mercury in the mouth was not commonly known. In recent times, non-metallic fillings have become more mainstream. It's worthwhile to research mercury poisoning in the *Physicians' Desk Reference*. I've had all my mercury removed and it helped me tremendously. See *Whole-Body Dentistry: Discover the Missing Piece to Better Health* by Mark A. Breiner.

Traveling to the Dead Sea in Israel, I met many other psoriasis patients. After this, I created a blog and website dedicated to communicating with these patients worldwide. In doing this, I've spoken with and shared stories with hundreds of other psoriasis patients during the past ten years. These new friends revealed a great deal of pain, embarrassment and shame associated with having acute psoriasis symptoms.

I now believe each of us can return home to our original state of health. We can greet our inner child and reclaim the sanity of our youth with our almost childlike stamina. It will, however, take time, courage, and a plan.

Do you think there is an easy, direct path to discover the way out of a health crisis? Don't we have to look deeper to uncover the original anatomical causes which may have led to a particular condition?

## THE PROCESS

I have successfully replicated a full clearing of my skin four separate summers, over the past decade, going for complete doctor supervised treatments at the Dead Sea. I want to share my process with you in a step by step manner.

In 2007, I went to the DMZ Medical Center at the Lot Hotel in Ein Bokek, Israel, for 28 days of psoriasis treatment. The DMZ clinic is a leading therapy center for many autoimmune conditions including psoriasis.

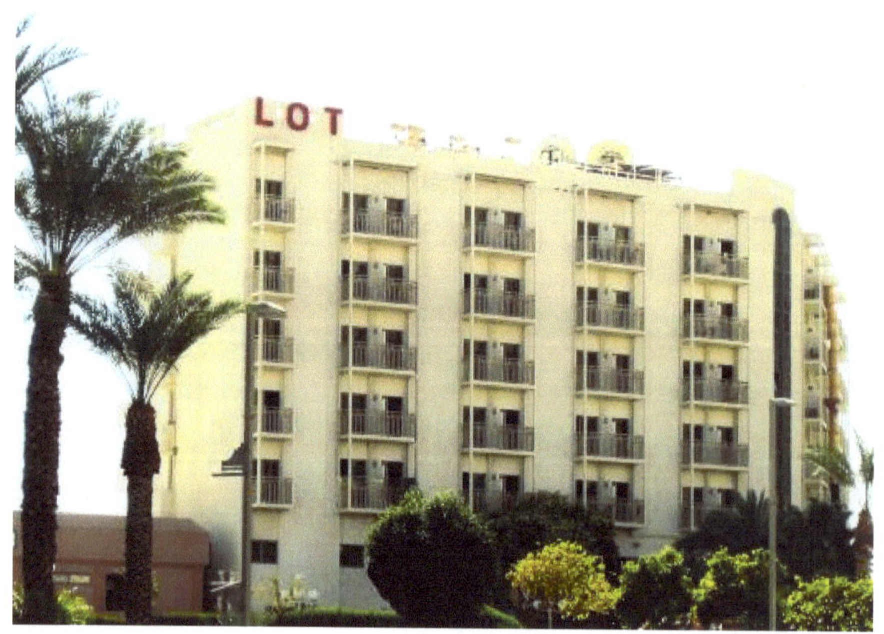


I really encourage an extended visit to the Dead Sea, if at all possible, because I feel that its water has a unique chemical makeup which when combined with the sun's healing qualities has enormous benefits. The water has been documented by dermatologists at this link - www.everydayhealth.com/psoriasis/treatment/can-dead-sea-salt-treat-psoriasis - to successfully treat psoriasis as a form of clearing and remission.

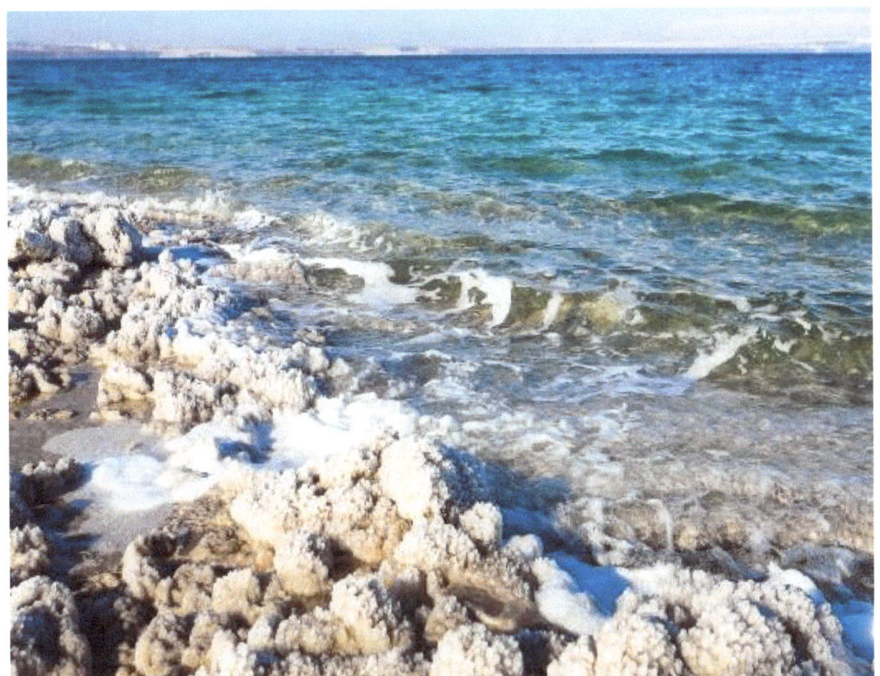

© Vvoe / Adobe Stock

While at the clinic, it became clear to me that by actually loving myself and taking care of all aspects of mind, physical body, and soul, I have been able to create a good healthy balance in life.

It is not advisable to try to do this entirely by yourself...but with the love and support of a team of qualified medical or natural health practitioners, so perhaps with these mentors, things may begin to happen in your own recovery. I know because it's happened this way for me and many others.

Come on this journey down a wonderful boardwalk. Visualize Israel's ancient salty sea with its amazing colored flowers and palm trees blowing in the extreme heat with waters reflecting against the nearby mountains.

**Accept the challenge**

I wonder how many of you readers would sojourn and live in this desert heat for a minimum of one month for such intense healing treatments? Thousands of patients from Europe, Russia, South Africa, South America, USA, Canada, and Australia have done exactly as I have for many years and each of them was forever changed.

After my first trip to the Dead Sea in 2007, I returned to the US with a strong yearning to share my healing experience with others. Initially, I posted a video on the internet and hundreds of people expressed interest in learning more about my treatment experience. A group of people joined me in 2013 when I led a trip to the DMZ clinic for four weeks.

I created a holistic and healing program including nutrition, relaxation, laughter and group meetings. The participants all bathed in the super salty water, breathed the mineral-rich air, and sat in the sweltering sun, day in and day out. Each of us returned home feeling great benefits. There are approximately 125 million people in the world with psoriasis and about 250 million with painful arthritis in their joints—comparable to the total population of the US. Ask them what they might be willing to do for even six months of calming and soothing relief from red skin, scales, pain, shame and suffering?

Brad (below) came with me in the summer of 2013 for six weeks of treatment. We practiced a healthy, low sugar, wheat and dairy free diet, and shared our stories of how and when psoriasis began for each of us. Brad had the worst skin condition I'd ever seen. His recovery experience was profound. By the end of treatment, he walked away experiencing remarkably clear skin for more than a year.

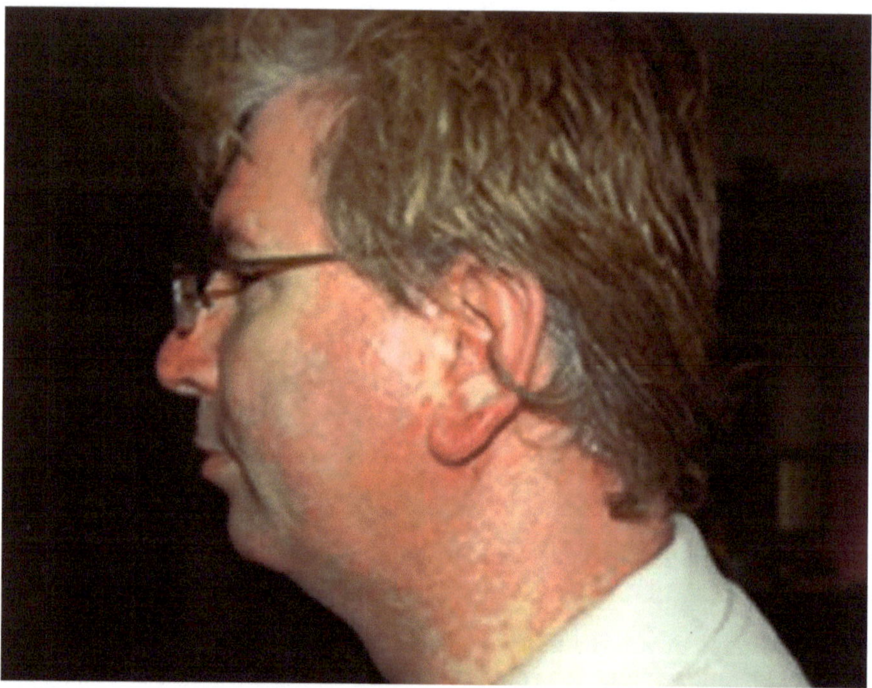

I offered him a structured program of nutrition, meditation, Qigong stretch, breathing and relaxation, plus funny movies and other laughter therapy. The combined treatment can be effective for all who stay the course of this healing journey. It has to do with calming the system to allow our body to become alkaline and less acid or toxic. Below, he is with his wife showing off his clear skin.

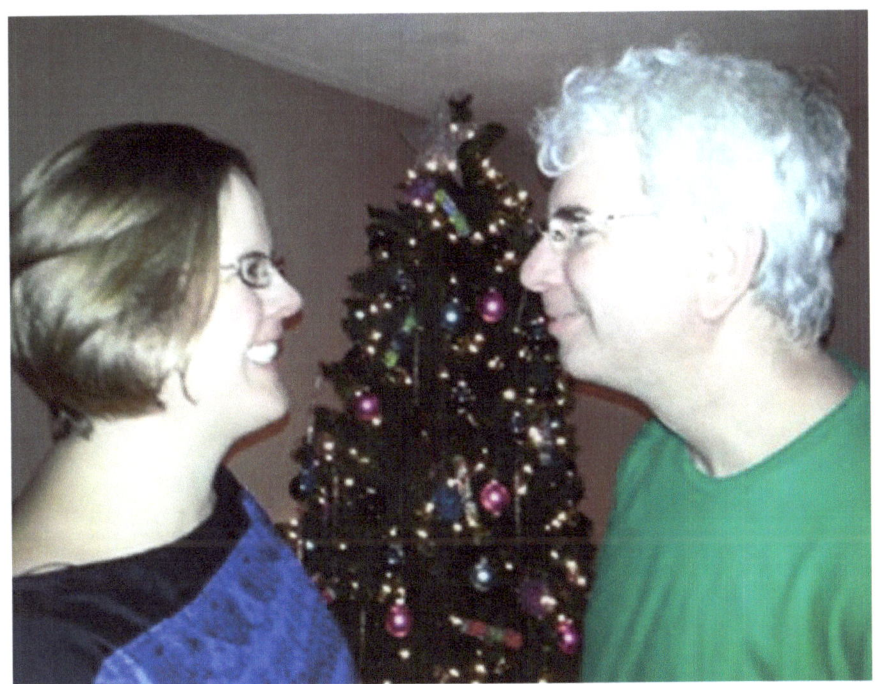



## COMPLIMENTARY SUPPORTS

For psoriasis patients, and many similar autoimmune conditions like arthritis, the journey begins here and now, with eating certain foods. Raw vs. cooked can matter, as well as the eating and chewing process. In the course of this journal and entire book, I will mention experts, their books and websites for you to study on your own—extracting ideas about what might be best for you. Remember it must be a personal choice and an "inside job" how you heal. The combination of nutrition, mind, body and spirit are all a part of the process in our healing.

How we chew, digest and eliminate properly is the next piece. How much stress we allow in our lives is another piece. How much exercise, regular and proper intimate sexual relations we enjoy, in mature loving relationships matters tremendously. Our DNA and our toxic environment can also tug at our homeostasis, the ability to balance and fight off old and new illness.

We are all constructed physiologically almost like other mammals with similar organs and perhaps even hearts and souls. This mind/body and spirit combination needs natural, non-toxic healthy nourishment. With the junk food industry of the last 70 years or so, all of this has been genetically altered, introducing many environmental pollutants, growth hormones, and toxic modifications which came with its processing and preservation. All designed to ship and feed people in stores elsewhere. Local production and selling became less common during these years of mass production.

Given thousands of natural plant-based substances to choose from, in the form they grow and are harvested, instead, since the 1950s, Westerners have sought instant pudding, and poor nutrition like processed white flour, bleached rice, homogenized milk and processed cheese which don't resemble what comes naturally from previously healthy fed cows and goats.

Never have so many people opted for fast food over a healthy salad grown in an organic garden. For centuries, our grandparents lived this way until we stopped taking the time to grow, prepare, chew and digest properly.

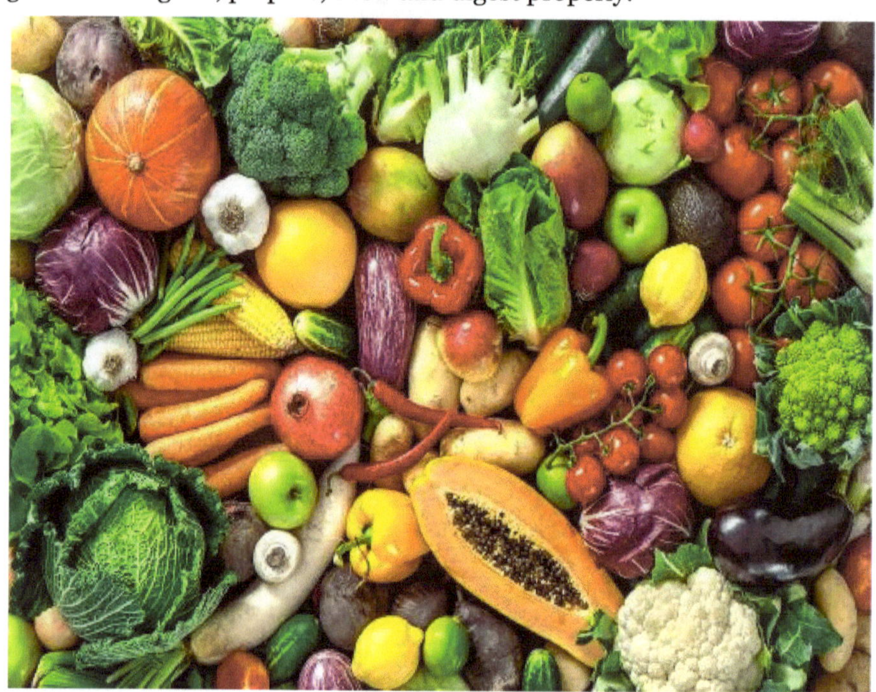

*The 5 Colors of Phytonutrients, © Alexander Raths / Adobe Stock*

This idea alone led me to create a nonprofit organization dedicated to this theme – HealthRightUSA began in 2007 after my initial Dead Sea treatment, but since changed to www.healthrightisrael.com to share what others in Israel are doing to help people heal naturally.

###

My mission and goal has been to write about and connect people with many safe healing modalities. Original readings in 2007 led me to world-famous nutritionists such as Dr. Joel Fuhrman with information at www.drfuhrman.com, author of the *Science of Skinny*, Dee McCaffrey at www.processedfreeamerica.org and T. Colin Campbell at www.whole.nutritionstudies.org. These great health activists and their organizations may also assist you in getting strong—to detox for a future life of health and longevity. We all can replenish and heal the source of life and primal energy within us, however, this is a very personal journey.

I have experienced that psoriasis appears as a skin condition but it is an autoimmune reaction due to a digestive problem. I also believe from speaking with experts that it is possible that the healing work needed will take longer than the patient can actually sustain. The longer the condition has been around the longer it may really take to reverse. We cannot claim any cure for everyone, but results for those who try a nutritional approach can greatly improve and be long lasting for many. This condition seems to afflict mostly Caucasians, with few known incidents among those of African descent, and currently millions of Asians. We can only surmise that it relates to an influx of Western foods worldwide.

Psoriasis has a lot of misery and mystery surrounding it. For the most part, acute cases are usually given very little hope for a successful cure by Western doctors.

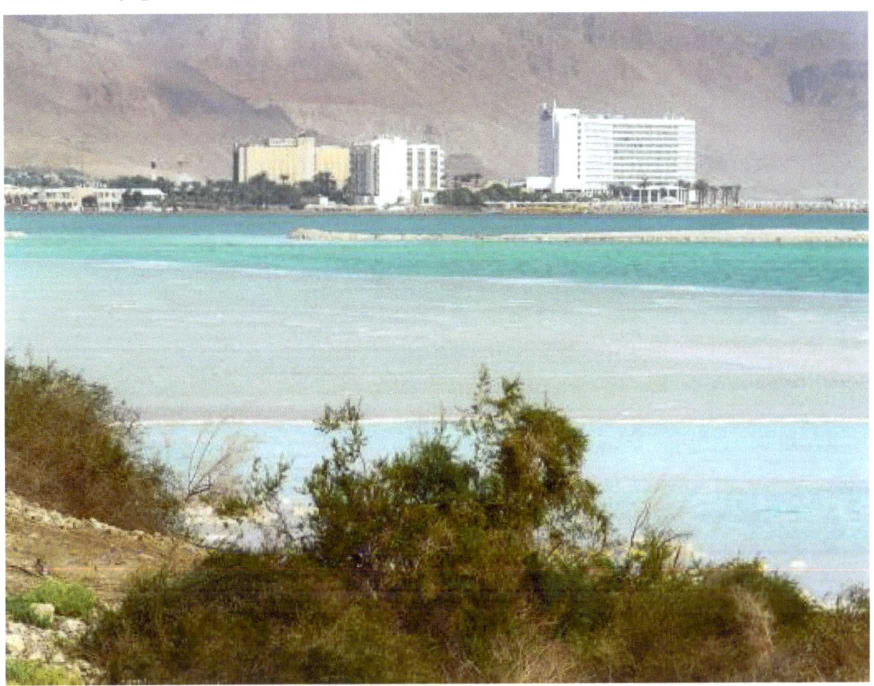

My story was written from 2007-17 and through this decade, the hope to help many readers in the future has sustained me. In 2013, I spent 81 days at the DMZ clinic during which time I gained insights into the healing process and became an experienced patient advocate.

My healing process involves extremely hard work using your entire mind, body and spiritual beliefs to bring on a complete change of lifestyle habits. I say this to you not as a doctor or a nurse, but instead, as a dedicated patient seeking natural relief for over 25 years.

In order for your remission to become long-lasting, these attitudes and behaviors must propel a shift in lifestyle. I learned from the clinicians at the DMZ that only 10% of the people who undergo this treatment stay in remission more than a year. What is it that these select few are doing better or differently?

Why don't more people remain clear-skinned over a longer period? It became clear to me there was no efficient way to properly track patients who did not return frequently. The clinic I have worked with only checks the skin remissions of people who actually do return. So, what happens to that missing group who may never return?

If you have been to the Dead Sea for this full three-week treatment and you have remained clear, please email me at mati@HealthRightIsrael.com to say what you have done which has helped you to remain more clear-skinned. Later I may be able to share this with others.

Perhaps patients don't do healthy things to maintain their new skin when they leave Israel and return to old bad health habits in their hometowns? Is it the toxic job, boss or even family member that keeps this individual from growing strong again? "Stress is a killer," they say, and how we handle all kinds of outside influences can cause great stress if not managed properly. This is why I use the idea of our gut in this discussion because people with high stress in life internalize their emotions and sickness in their organs. I have certainly been guilty of this.

It will take at least three to four weeks to get relaxed and motivated enough to return home with a committed goal. Remaining free of psoriasis, after you are cleared of all redness and lesions, is possible. It's up to us to keep healthy and positive in every way.

I began talking about my journey to Israel's *Sea of Life*, as the Black Hebrews of Dimona call it, the lowest spot on the planet, known for its relaxing detoxing, healing mineral waters, unique air and sun rays. And, I believe there is no other natural medicinal location quite like it. Now we can agree it is not "dead."

Below are my own pictures of acute psoriasis healing (before and after shots) during that same summer. You can see a change in only 18 days.

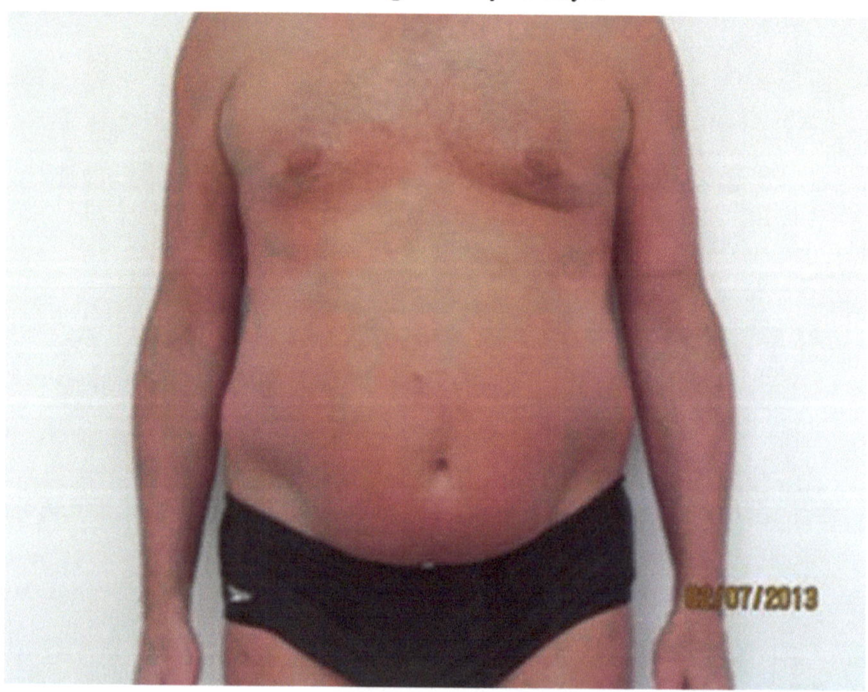

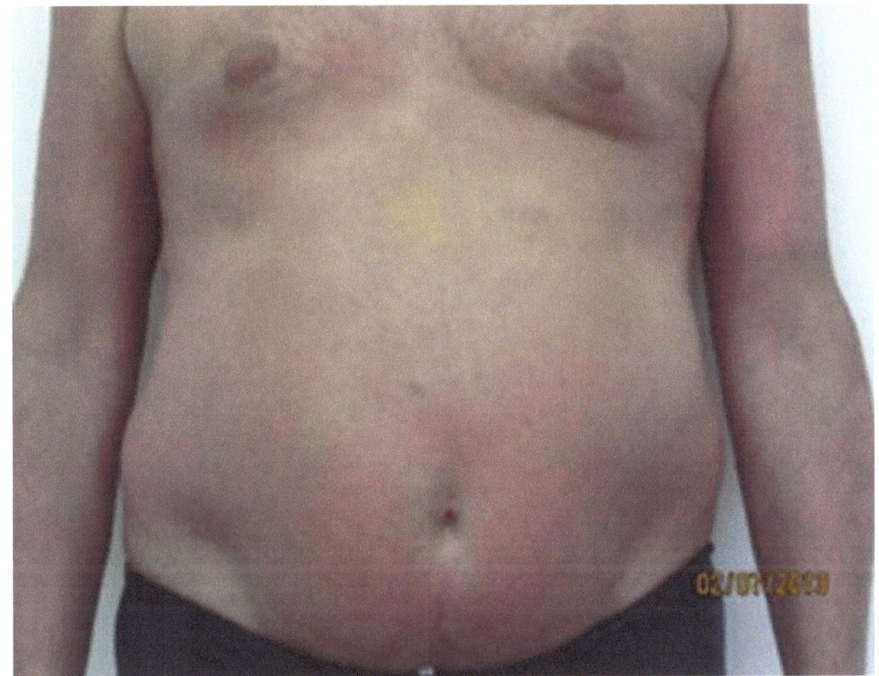

As all patients travel through this process of clearing, they return through the proverbial "eye of the needle." To heal, we must travel through this zone, metaphorically, psychologically and even physiologically, as we find our way back home to the original full health of our childhood.

For some, it's a process of uncovering traumas of our past childhood, which may have adversely affected our health. It can be done by anyone with persistence, by activating a plan to undo this damage. Much of our health is literally in our guts—regarding digestion. It will take time, money and a huge desire to restore inside gut health.

Here is a video of myself at **https://tinyurl.com/yb8t74xw** on the nutrition and attitude program I created along with Dead Sea treatments, sun, creams and medical consultations. This video clip is a time-lapse of daily progress while dipping in the waters and sunning my skin. During this first stay, at this amazingly restful and hot spot on the planet, I began to have the full belief that I could succeed.
I kept the following journal entries so readers could see my daily thoughts and progress. Please don't skip the reading process, however, because it's the journey that really counts, not the destination.

## ACKNOWLEDGMENTS

In thinking about how grateful I am that I was able to afford this first journey of healing initially at the age of 53, I want to express my unbridled appreciation to my wife Ronni for her unlimited belief in my abilities to change, her undying respect and unconditional love for me. Many times since then I have felt undeserving and not able to show her my gratitude. This is one of the areas of thanks I need to offer her unconditionally and repeatedly.

Also, I have an unwavering belief in a loving G-d which I discovered alone in Italy while emotionally confused in my 19th year. I was seeking guidance at this turning point in life when I experienced a strong intense light. Now I know it was His Truth, that of an infinite loving G-d. While in Israel, during frequent visits, I have felt this exact same strong warm light each time as I've healed my skin.

To you, the reader or patient, I'm stepping out on faith that you are also on a journey or a quest for personal healing in finding your own truth. Are you open to the notion that we are players in altering our own healing path? Can you see we are made in the image of an awesome G-d?

Therefore, this literally means we have some of His attributes:

—The power of the spoken word (creation)

—The ability to be artistic and creative (designing what will be)

—The ability to show love and caring about others (including giving us the potential to bear children to care for)

As I reflect back on these lessons learned, "in the image of G-d" signifies that we can speak what we want, design how we live, love and care about people. But before any of this can happen there is one cardinal rule which must be obeyed.

"Love thy neighbor as thyself." Now this is the toughest of all concepts in both the Old Bible (the Jewish Torah) and New Bible (Christian Testaments). Why is this process so difficult for the average person to accomplish?

As patients with symptoms of psoriasis, redness, often we battle with this idea of lacking self-love. So many of the other people I met in the treatment clinic at the Dead Sea were not happy with themselves. They were angry and felt victimized by this skin condition.

Through much soul-searching, I have gleaned that in order to "love thy neighbor as thyself," I first had to love myself. Essentially, I had been inadvertently breaking this cardinal rule in life...I sincerely don't believe I was loving myself yet. And, in this way, I was avoiding the ancient lessons of caring for others properly as I was so preoccupied with my own suffering.

Wow! This blew me away. For years I didn't possess the self-confidence to say *I did love who I was.* Even today, I am often critical of myself and beat myself up. Guess what? I have resolved that this belief must stop. We all can no longer dislike or on the extreme side, hate ourselves. In fact, in reading the Dalai Lama's (see below, youthful Tibetan monk showing this kind of unconditional love) comments in his book *The Art of Happiness*, it became evident that in his culture, the concept of self-abasement is unheard of. They just don't understand it.

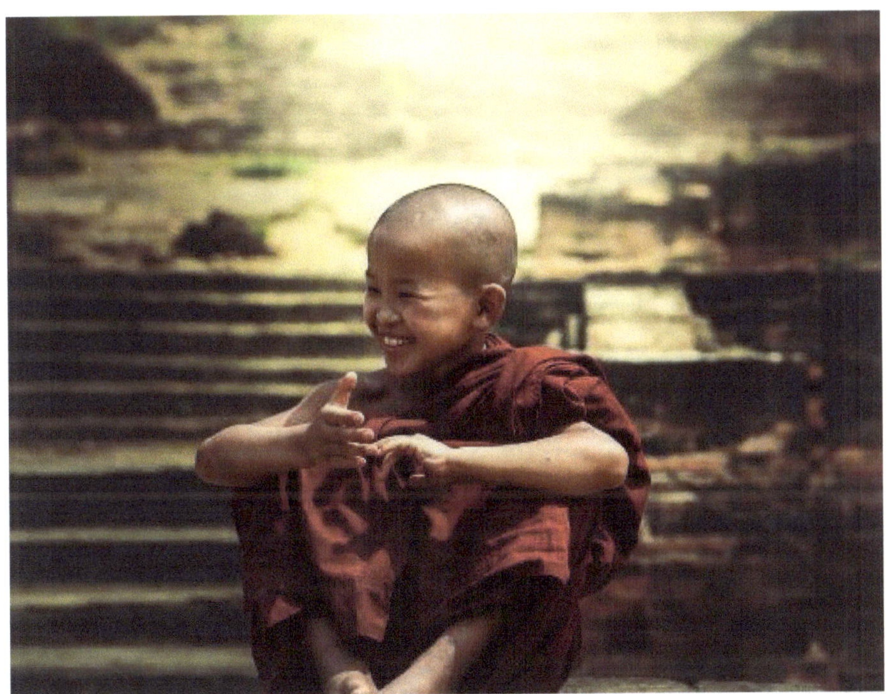



In Western society, we hurt ourselves on a regular basis by:

—Smoking cigarettes which we know can cause cancer.

—Driving drunk where we can kill people, often the other driver or our innocent passengers.

—Excessively taking over-the-counter drugs or those which we know are illegal making us sick or worse.

—Overeating and not exercising as we know we should.

The reason why I'm saying this is to open the reader to the idea of starting a process of loving thyself. Allow it, just love and not judge anyone else. This will begin the inner healing needed to succeed in any deep and permanent healing program.

We can do this day-by-day. It's best to remove yourself from all stresses in your current environment. This is why a trip to Israel's warm and dry Dead Sea is a wonderful solution. There you will find healing waters, sun that melts away your red and flaky skin lesions easily. It's not just a vacation but a relaxing return to that special innocent childhood zone you once had, and perhaps, may have lost. Here, at the lowest hot spot on Earth you'll again become yourself. For three to four glorious weeks it will feel great and you will think of no one else, just as it should be. You can start loving yourself deeply. It's not selfish, it's absolutely vital. It's a true leap of faith...

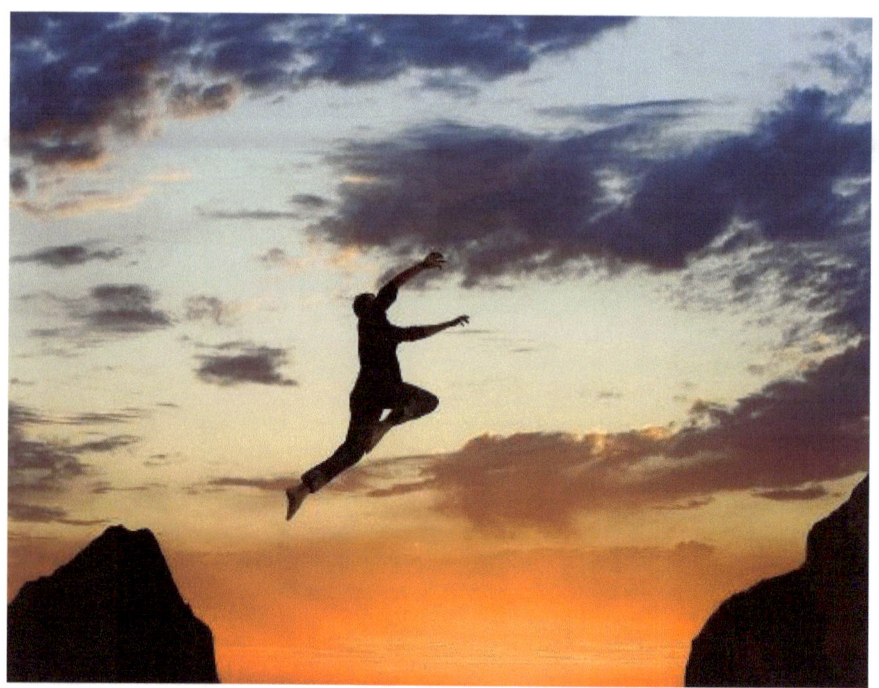



Now we must begin the work at hand. It is not a battle to overcome illness, as many see it. It is an act of love, laughter, eating less, stretching more, breathing better, listening more to others and to your inner self. Indeed, it's simply a leap of faith into that which is unseen. It's believing again, as we did in childhood, that we can again be innocent, clear in our heart, mind and trust that our skin can smooth out as well.

I assure you of one thing. Your healing will not follow my plan exactly since we are all unique biological and multi-billion-dollar masterpieces. No two people are identical in DNA composition or structure.

What I'm proposing is a plan which requires taking a full three to four weeks of your life as a gift for your health and longevity. It's a common belief that to make a lasting change in lifestyle direction it requires a minimum of 21-days in a row to break any habit and form a new one.

It is a real, honest commitment to change your lifestyle habits and then to follow-through in your own unique way when you return to your hometown. What you will take from this process should allow you to return home and make a very new life. With this agreement to change, you may see the results you hope for.

Only you can be the judge of this. Einstein and others have said, "If you do what you've always done, you'll get what you've always got." Why repeat old, unhealthy mistakes. Please don't let this be your future. Healing is a decision to sincerely change.

Love yourself as I love you, without even meeting you. I'm capable of loving who I am, in spite of my many mistakes in the past. I'm better for them. Don't judge anyone or yourself because we can all move ahead to a better place, a better world.

## Preparation for the journey

**June 29, 2007** – One month prior to my departure for healing at the Dead Sea, I began a liver cleanse diet recommended by Dr. Jennifer Botwick, my USA naturopath. I want to give credit also to my naturopath in Israel, Dr. Avraham Moskowitz (read more at www.healthrightisrael.com/healing-with-food-exercise-and-mindfulness about his philosophy) from Jerusalem who consulted with my group in the 2013 session.

Below is the liver cleansing program I did for six days with the guidance of Dr. Botwick before leaving the USA, just to experience good digestion and elimination. The following are the ingredients:

- —1 onion, peeled and chopped
- —1 head of cabbage, chopped
- —2 cloves of garlic, peeled and chopped
- —2 carrots, chopped
- —2 celery stalks, trimmed and chopped
- —1 bunch of parsley, chopped
- —5 kale leaves, chopped
- —2 sheets of nori seaweed vegetable, chopped
- —4 pieces of okra, trimmed and chopped
- —1 cup of uncooked brown rice
- —1 pinch of Braggs amino acids
- —2 quarts of filtcrcd watcr

Combine all ingredients into a large soup pot and simmer over a low heat for 1.5 hours. Eat warmed-up as often as you are hungry for a maximum of six days. During this time, I never felt hungry. I had good and regular bowel movements. It truly felt like the food preparation was cleaning out my insides.

During day one of this program I experienced a very restful Sabbath. I felt no hunger and enjoyed the food. I added rice cakes to give myself something crunchy. I also made my own spread out of celery, garlic, ochre and olive oil blended into a puree. It was pungent and divine. In addition, I made Chinese detox tea consisting of these herbs: dandelion, burdock and echinacea roots.

In Eastern medicine, it is commonly known that the liver is a major organ in dealing with toxins in the body and it may be dysfunctional in psoriasis patients. In recent readings, I have noted that the liver can be connected with anger and indignation.

Interesting, no? Also, other organs such as kidneys are associated with emotions of thought and contemplation as well as hearing and understanding. Lastly our spleen connects with our laughter and exuberance and gallbladder delves into our levels of touch and sexuality.

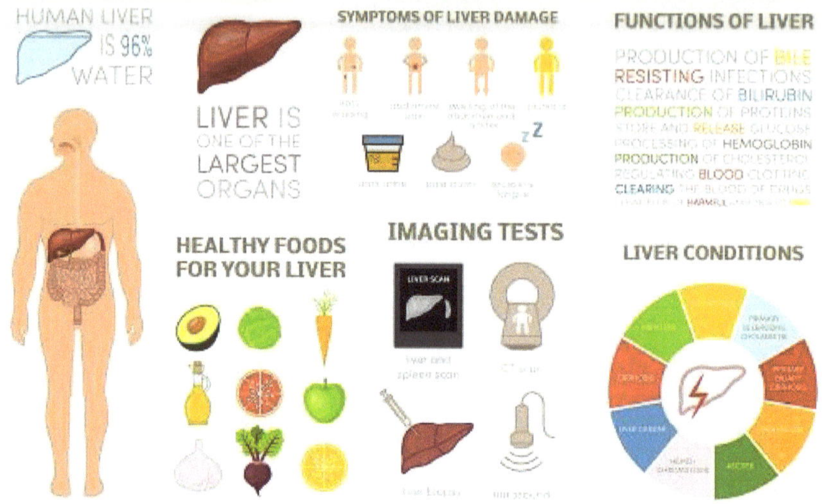


*© Marina_ua / Adobe Stock*

So, what does this all infer about our healing process? If we can optimize, cleanse and restore these organs to allow for better flow and healing, then it makes sense we could improve ways in which we:

—Temper our anger and indignation

—Contemplate becoming more elevated

—Become less self-absorbed

—Allow ourselves heartfelt joy, laughter to be youthful again

—Enjoy touching and sexuality to be open and free with our soul mate

—Rebuild confidence, pride (lack of shame), a more positive mental attitude

—Focus on our job, relax and create an ease (lack of frustration)

As I would be departing for the Dead Sea clinic in exactly one month, in preparation, I shaved my face, chest and head to begin suntanning all of me, right down to my bathing suit.

**June 30, 2007** – In the evening, I went to the beach, near my Connecticut home, to get some late day sunrays. My plan was to begin a slow tan without burning. The cleansing diet above continued well. I was instructed by my doctor to slowly begin reintroducing a few other foods, one-by-one, at the end of the cleansing process. We both wanted to see if I would experience any allergic reactions.

In the process of researching other ways to do self-guided nutrition, my wife referred me to www.doctoryourself.com where I found a useful protocol for fish oils, vegetable juice fasting, zinc supplements with vitamin B-2, B-3, A, C, and/or a good multivitamin.

Along with a booklet called *Psoriasis Can Be Cured* by Dr. Robert E. Connolly, I used all of this new information to begin developing my individualized nutrition plan during and after my stay in Israel. I decided I must really believe in my own healing if I was to become successful. I had no idea what the results would really be. Many of the items on my nutrition list can be found in Dr. Connolly's book.

In addition, during the month prior to departure, I began reading books about healing and positive mental powers, such as:

    —*The Art of Happiness* by the Dalai Lama

    —*Healing and the Power of the Mind* by Dr. Andrew Weil

    —*Timeless Healing, The Power and Biology of Belief* by Herbert Benson, M.D. and his earlier work, *The Relaxation Response, a Simple Meditative Technique that will Unlock Your Hidden Assets.*

    —*When All You've Ever Wanted Isn't Enough* by Rabbi Harold Kushner

    —*Why People Don't Heal and How They Can* by Caroline Myss, Ph.D.

These works along with meditation tapes, music, prayer and exercise were my process for getting into the proper state of mind, a zone of healing, before and during my stay at the clinic in Israel. I cannot speak highly enough about these books which are also in some cases available on audio. So, search online and you may get these gems or others just as good.

Please don't try to skip through the tulips. You must pay now or pay later. Dig in and read. Dog-ear the books, yes, own them. Use a yellow highlighter, and write notes, perhaps even write your own journal like this one. Why not? Send it to me and I'll read yours too.

**August 2, 2007** – At last, I arrived at the Dead Sea, jet-lagged…and a bit unsure if this was really the right place for me, after all of this long-range planning. I needed a few days to acclimate myself to the extreme dry heat. That first day, I soon met the head nurse and later my personal doctor at the DMZ clinic. It was reassuring to know they had seen many others who had 80% skin psoriasis, as bad as mine. I wanted the truth about the possibility of improvement vs. a complete cure. It was late Thursday in Israel. Still unsure, with many things unresolved, I fell asleep into a deep surreal and dreamlike state. As I faded…*Was I finally in Israel? Would I heal?*

**August 3, 2007** – That Friday morning when I arrived, I spoke with a Russian nurse who needed a translator. The secretary who translated, explained things and they both gave me the protocol (below) describing what I needed to do in daylight hours, as I began my gradual healing. Observe how much time I would spend daily in the sea and sun during my special medical treatments for psoriasis. I cannot emphasize enough how rigorous and exacting this process needed to be to avoid being sunburnt or getting a sunstroke while seeking the optimal healing treatment for my skin lesions. The doctor at the clinic later explained to me that this was a 25-30-year research protocol that he and his staff had arrived at. Each patient at this clinic needed their own evaluation, then a customized version of this chart prior to beginning a treatment in the hot desert sun and sea.

The schedule describes how often I had to go to the Dead Sea (durations) and when to sunbathe. In addition, there was a unique combination of creams that I will not go into, as this is the trademark of the doctor and nurse at the clinic. The precise use and frequency of sun/sea treatments depends on each patient's severity, type of lesions and pigmentation.

| Day number | Dead Sea in "shade" area under gazebo | Sunlight in solarium for entire body | Number of cycles per day |
| --- | --- | --- | --- |
| 1 | 5 minutes | 10 minutes | 2 times |
| 2 | 5 minutes | 15 minutes | 2 times |
| 3 | 5 minutes | 20 minutes | 2 times |
| 4 | 5 minutes | 15 minutes | 3 times |
| 5 | 5 minutes | 20 minutes | 3 times |
| 6 | 5 minutes | 20 minutes | 3 times |
| 7 | 10 minutes | 30 minutes | 3 times |
| 8 | 10 minutes | 30 minutes | 3 times |
| 9 | 10 minutes | 40 minutes | 3 times |
| 10 | 10 minutes | 40 minutes | 3 times |
| 11 | 10 minutes | 40 minutes | 3 times |
| 12 | 10 minutes | 40 minutes | 4 times |
| 13 | 15 minutes | 40 minutes | 4 times |
| 14 | 15 minutes | 40 minutes | 4 times |
| 15 | 15 minutes | 40 minutes | 4 times |
| Repeat | This | Level | Forward! |

*Schedule of sea and sunlight treatments from the clinic*

**August 4, 2007** – Having adjusted to the new time zone and my surroundings, I began to ask myself why I had ventured forth on this expensive, risky and unknown venture. I had researched that 97% of the patients who went to the Dead Sea had major or complete healing—which convinced me to fully commit to this adventure.

While it has never been a life-threatening illness, psoriasis has been annoying and embarrassing while swimming at every summer beach...with all eyes glaring at me in disgust. Nonetheless, I knew it would be a relief to me, my wife, and family if I could eliminate this upsetting and stigmatizing condition.

My thoughts rambled on...*how could I complain or make a big thing over this illness which most doctors said could not be cured?* Especially since I've been blessed in all other ways with a wonderful family; my beautiful wife Ronni of over 30 years, my three gorgeous and talented daughters Alexandra (who has a wonderful daughter of her own now), Hannah and Sophia who brighten each day of my existence on this troubled planet.

So why was I so ready to leave my wonderful family for a month and make an expensive investment of over $6,000 to deal with this skin ailment in such an intense way? My tendency, throughout my youth, and going forward into adult life, had been to go "all-out" at everything.

For example, as a child of ten, I built my own photography studio soon after I was given a camera and some developing supplies by my great-uncle Morris. He encouraged me to make my own prints and enlargements as he once had. I wanted to be like him, an independent man who'd traveled the world, took pictures and videos of many cultures and places. See, I was always looking for a mentor, a role model of sorts.

At the age of 14, I saw a potter throw a clay vessel on a wheel at a museum in Brooklyn, and within months I'd built my own potter's wheel and became an apprentice to master potters in Mexico, Maine and later in Italy. Clearly, no moss collected on me.

I always threw my whole self into each new idea and venture. Just like in pottery I guess, literally and figuratively one must "throw" clay to make a vessel. So as profound as this may sound, I was forming a "new" Matthew Allen vessel.

In recent years, I became a high school math teacher, and while this was rewarding in terms of helping kids learn a tough subject like mathematics, it became the most challenging experience of my life, beyond raising our own daughters. Kids are very needy, and I longed for a chance to help, maybe even teach/coach adults. Perhaps this new direction of health and wellness would be a fit for me as I moved into the next healing phase of my personal life. Who knew?

### Reflections after fourth treatment at the Dead Sea

Now, at 64, I look back and wonder about the meaning of many things. I don't question my marriage and having children. They are the greatest blessing I could ever have, to personally enjoy them and leave a vibrant family as a legacy beyond myself. I do often wonder what it must be like for people without children in their old age. To whom do they turn?

The real question now, however, is what am I doing beyond my family for the good of mankind? Can I take this challenge of healing myself and turn it into something worthwhile and meaningful for others who also face psoriasis and have not succeeded in healing this difficult condition alone?

In reading Rabbi Kushner's *When All You've Ever Wanted Isn't Enough*, I must comment that all I have ever wanted is truly enough, I just haven't reached certain desired achievements yet. In many ways, I feel very fortunate that I am a late bloomer and that G-d has, in his infinite wisdom, allowed me to achieve family success first so I might spend the rest of my years creating a healthy life for others to follow. But for this to be true, I must become the leader. No more talk. Right? I must complete the task I set out to finish in 2007, to be a survivor who has completely healed psoriasis.

I have given my love to my children and wife so that they always know I'm there. While I may not make a monetary fortune, we have always been blessed with love, closeness and have had the necessities of life. Now, I feel obliged to show my children, by example, how we must find a way to give opportunities to others, empower them, show them to "how to fish." My plans going forward are to teach others healthy nutritional survival skills for living a full life and perhaps ways to help them make a good living.

People are always looking for ways to improve. They are also looking for leaders. I'm a born leader and cannot spend any more of my life hiding as a follower in a bureaucratic system like teaching. I'm ready for my next major "give-back" direction.

During 2013, I became committed to the world of natural healing and wellness. I discovered that some people resisted their own treatment if it meant going all the way with diet, nutrition and positive actions. This may sound strange, but when you read about a concept called Woundology Theory in *Why People Don't Heal and How They Can* by Caroline Myss, Ph.D., this may make a lot more sense.

I want you to visualize that you absolutely can clear your skin, starting at the Dead Sea and with diet, exercise and by embracing the process of self-love.

The steps are:

1. Dead Sea treatment

2. Relaxation, meditation, laughter, exercise

3. Nutrition to cleanse the body of toxins

The challenge we all face is that when we fall down or someone pushes us down in life, sometimes we hate ourselves or beat ourselves up for failing. This is a downward spiral that some people go to their grave replaying. I know, because I have been caught in this depressing role. Getting out of it is a matter of self-love and self-talk. We must tell ourselves we are worthy of more and start over with a renewed spirit.

To win in our own game of life, we must stop self-abasement and climb out of the hole fighting back with love. Being a victim and not a victor is a losing battle. That is what reading about and avoiding *Woundology Theory* teaches us to do. So, I suggest you read the entire book by Caroline Myss.

## Returning to the 2007 journal

**August 5, 2007** – Today I met my doctor to get further instructions on how to use the Dead Sea in conjunction with the sun treatments. He was very easy to talk with and explained the program in great detail. Answering many questions, clarifying what results I should expect to see, he promised to help me heal my skin, at least for the near term. I smiled in gratitude.

First, he examined how badly I needed the treatment and confirmed I was 80% inflicted with psoriasis. Then he told me people who do the entire program for three to four weeks see great improvement and many are in remission for up to six to eight months. Some return for yearly tune-ups to help healing to continue. And most people who returned two to three times in five years were able to go into a more complete remission.

While my doctor was dedicated to working on my topical skin condition, in my heart, I believed I needed internal healing, as well. A principal of Eastern medicine and homeopathy/naturopathy guides us to listen to our organs and meridians (pathways in the body connecting vital energy) using teas, breathing, Qigong exercises and joy. I really do resonate with these beliefs.

**August 8, 2007** – In this entry, I will mention a few of the things which have made a great difference in the past few days, but I will lead with a book discussion referencing *When All You've Ever Wanted Isn't Enough* by Kushner. I won't describe books in too much detail because that is for you to dig in and discover. In this text, however, I wish to point out the essence of his writing as it relates to healing psoriasis, living in the moment, peaceful coexistence in the world, and mentorship.

I see how I must learn to rejoice in the moment more. Living for now is paramount to lowering stress, gaining strength and health.

Walking through the streets of Jerusalem on the Sabbath, I experienced something I read in Rabbi Kushner's book. In 2014-16 we lived in Israel as a family and my middle daughter used to laugh at me. I would be talking about tonight, tomorrow or some other distant concept with the family on a Friday night. My darling Hannah just said to me, "Daddy, stop thinking so much. Look up. Then, look down. Look to your back, and then to your front. Look from side to side. Now, just breathe." Guess what? She was not telling, but actually showing me how to live in G-d's gift, the present or the now, in order to be present and to not waste a special moment preaching about something that hasn't occurred yet, probably isn't even so important, especially not on our holy Sabbath. What a terrific gift and lesson. I am always grateful to have received this from her.

I appreciate what I have, who I am now and literally rejoice as in the concept of "eat, drink and be merry!" In addition to not getting lost in the past or projecting into the future, I must truly avoid feelings of jealousy about what others possess, any selfishness about what I might possess, or lack of trust in people. This is not to say, don't be careful amongst strange cultures or neighborhoods we visit infrequently, but, in general I must develop an open, honest, generous and cheerful attitude. Call it our *karma* needed in order to restore health and maintain this positive approach to live each day fully.

During the three to four weeks you may spend healing at the Dead Sea clinic you will experience a wonderfully concentrated time to truly digest ideas, books, and of course, healthy foods. I will also say that, in this time and space of healing, you may encounter the most remarkable, honest and courageous people you've ever met, provided you are open to sharing your mutual challenges with psoriasis.

Rabbi Kushner talks about how the plant and animal kingdom coexist so that they all find a place to grow and endure (p. 183). In thinking about this, in the summer of 2007, I could not help but worry about the fighting in Iraq and the many wars in the Middle East over religion and oil wells. I wondered, *why couldn't people be as sophisticated as plants and animals?*

Kushner also talks (p. 170) about the importance of true mentorship in our civilized world. We not only need good teachers to guide us through life, but we must learn enough to become ongoing guides and mentors to the next generation. We should all strive to have a positive impact on others in our lifetime.

He goes on to say this kind of generative lifestyle of making a difference in the lives of others is actually what keeps one healthy and living longer. Even if we do die younger, while helping others, we have actually served G-d much more having loved and lived with a purpose.

Kushner (p. 162) asks each of us to think about what are some of the non-negotiable elements of our lives. What must we have in order to feel fulfilled? Here are the main thoughts I gleaned from this chapter.

Kushner claims we must realize that pain and struggle are built into life. He continues to assert that we need to allow ourselves to belong to a community. Finally, he concludes that we must experience and acknowledge that we have made a mark and our lives therefore have meaning. Rabbi Kushner ends his book by praying that we each have progeny to further bless the world, that we plant a tree that provides fruit and shade for others, and lastly, try to write a book to share thoughts and spirit as a legacy.

It's evident we are only here for a relatively short "bleep" on the radar screen, compared to the Omnipresent and Eternal One. When Rabbi Kushner talked about being a *mensch*, it really hit home because I know this is the area I want to move toward in my healing. (*Mensch* is a Yiddish word for a very kind person who gives to others unconditionally, and like my father, is loved dearly for this.) Only a few people stood out in my past as having achieved this. My dad, Arthur (below), was one. He always made people feel good and we were sad when he left the room. Indeed, we were each crushed when he left our lives at the relatively young age of 75 after his battle with leukemia.

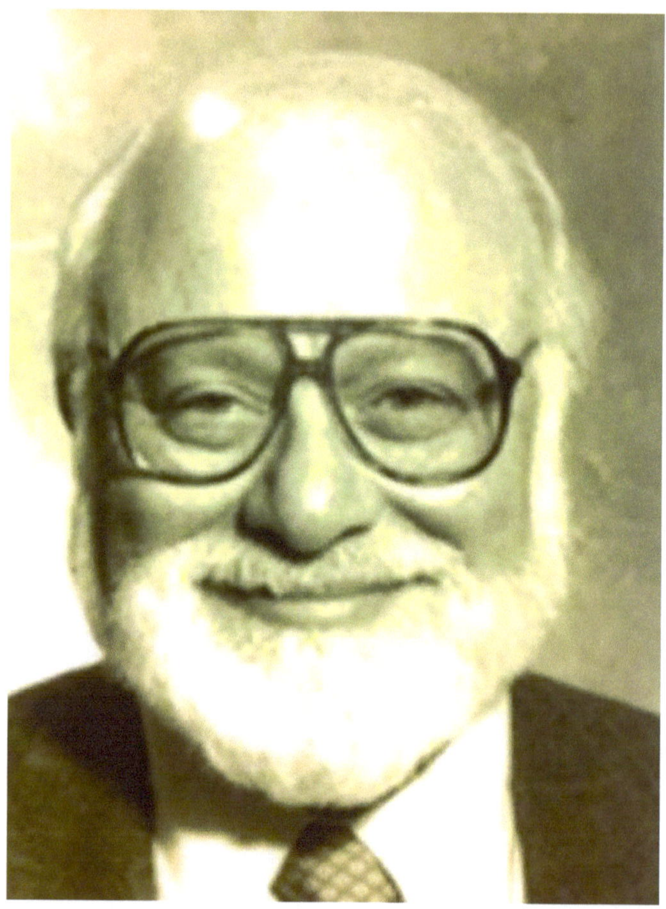

I think about this special trait—being happy, fulfilled and sharing this with others. I wonder how in my 60s, I can begin to become the person who is present and attentive to others, someone others expect will bring joy and not sadness. This easygoing style of breathing in and out only positive energy, learning and sharing, gives rise to the kind of healthy lifestyle I've been missing.

It's ironic, but I'm now capable of becoming more like someone who I've admired all these years...my own dad. I've spent so many years being sincerely afraid to outdo him, only to realize finally that this was not really possible. Once I began to visualize how he had an incredible way with people, I admired him so much more. He simply made them happy to be alive. All of this came through in his smile. At last, in my sixth decade, I wish to become more like him.

Now, I want to spend the rest of my years getting to know people on their terms—without my personal agenda. I am grateful to Rabbi Kushner for this extremely valuable lesson.

**August 10, 2007** – Today was a great day. After my eighth day of going in the sea and sun multiple times, I noticed a major clearing. I could really see, at this early point, how I would be clearing totally by the end of two to three weeks. Finally, it was evident it could actually happen this fast—by my fourth week in treatment.

With this great new feeling of optimism, I began to mellow and decided to incorporate giving myself a time each day for built-in meditation, prayer and relaxation. In keeping with the theme of relaxation, my next reading was Dr. Herbert Benson's *The Relaxation Response* which made me laugh and think I would be ready for yoga or a Pilates class when I returned home. If not, however, I felt convinced I could find at least 20 minutes twice each day to elicit what Dr. Benson calls the Relaxation Response.

These days, I use this video at **https://tinyurl.com/y7hxvc7h** to practice Qigong special meridian and organ healing moves. It helps me breathe and relax as I begin every day, no matter where I am. I just need my lightweight tablet and Wi-Fi. I suggest doing this early and/or late each day for just ten minutes. It could make a difference, helping us all to relax, heal and meditate.

Before I go into any of the details I learned about the Relaxation Response process, I must say that the book includes a great technical discussion about what happens to the brain under stress and things in our life which may cause it. We know how we each live with stress and that it's a great contributor to the condition we label as psoriasis (p. 74).

Dr. Benson tells how each religion and culture has had a way to reach this zone of healthy breathing and relaxation. Whether it's through eastern yoga, transcendental meditation, hypnosis, traditional prayer, breathing exercises, etc., clearly, you can find a modality that works for you. You'll see what relates to you on a personal level. I've gravitated toward Jewish prayer. Simply substitute a single syllable mantra of your choosing and try this same method yourself.

Dr. Benson gives very specific instructions for how the Relaxation Response is to work (p. 115). Be comfortable, focus on silence, relax muscles, breathe naturally, don't worry about doing it right. Continue for 10-15 minutes, give yourself this time, mostly with your eyes closed. At the end, wait before you stand to regain balance.

I am able to utilize our Jewish prayer as a partial mantra. For example, in the morning and afternoon we say, "Hear oh Israel, L-rd our G-d the L-rd is One!" at least two to three times a day during the week and on the Sabbath. (In the Jewish faith, some choose to hyphenate the name of the Almighty as it's only to be written or spoken in actual prayer, not in discussions of this nature.) It's a very useful repetition when you take the last two words in *Shemah Isroel* (the Hebrew version), *Hashem Elokanu, Hashem e-cHod.* (*Hashem* means the "Name" and is okay to write or speak outside of prayers.)

With practice, the Relaxation Response should come with little effort. Practice the technique once or twice daily, but not within two hours following a meal because it may interfere with our digestive processes.

Using my personal mantra from Jewish prayers I simply, breathe in and out, saying "One" in and "One" out, repetitively. So in Hebrew, I just say *eh* with the in breath and *cHod* with the out breath. It means G-d is One which I enjoy saying. It gives me peace. I can do this at the morning and evening service seven days a week and achieve my 20-minute Relaxation Response to help relax and heal my skin. I have read that it might also assist in lowering or preventing high blood pressure.

My general goal is to use this as a part of my daily prayer process to help me become calm, address stress more easily and not allow my skin to return to a psoriatic state. I also wish and plan that my life be extended with this practice.

**August 13, 2007, midnight** – Unable to sleep and restless. I was pondering why some people get psoriasis and others do not. I got up with a Eureka moment and started developing my ideas to help myself reverse my own condition. During my stay at the Dead Sea, every psoriasis patient I spoke with was aware of their own personal triggers which began psoriasis lesions. After all, no one I spoke with was born with psoriasis and they realized something caused their condition.

Many of us realized it was stress related. I wondered, *what flipped the switch for all of us?* It seemed, across the board, we all had some unique emotional trauma which drove us into a sadness resulting in this condition. Something just may have snapped!

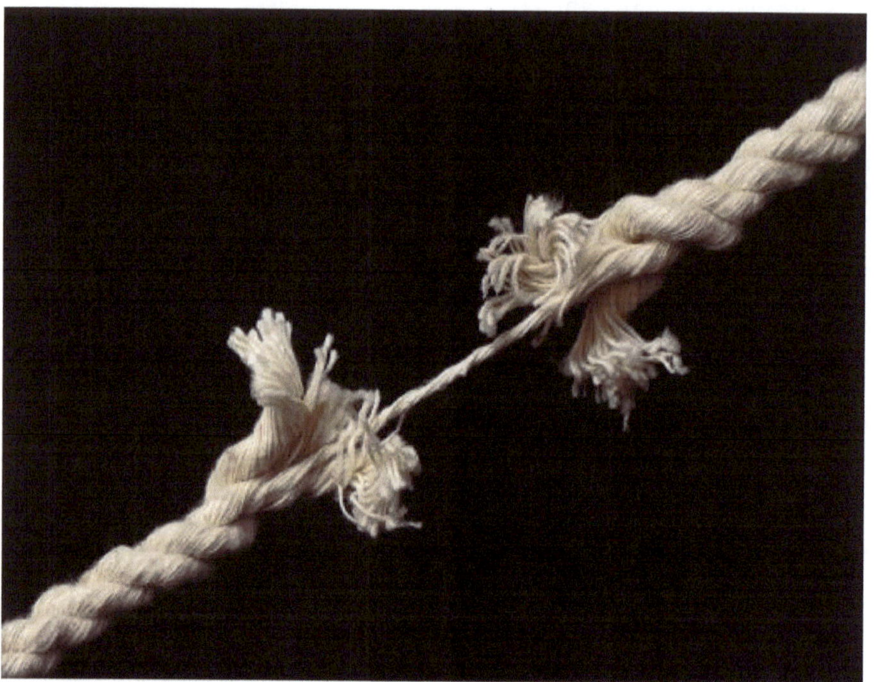

© *Dmitry Knorre / Adobe Stock*

I believe each of us has a biologically similar exterior but our individual traumas were unique to each of us. An analogy would be a burglar cracking open a locked safe with tons of money inside...only we as individuals have that unique combination of numbers to dial and get inside to release our own trauma. In my thinking, however, I feel that once I get inside, I must remove those unhealthy feelings to successfully heal my skin.

With all of the soul-searching I've done, there are three basic concepts or processes which may effectively open my personal safe and free me of this disease:

 1. Separation

 2. Letting go

 3. Forgiving

As I see these words, I'm sure they are mine because I want to cry! I struggle still with why I cannot cry about all of this yet. I want to open up and let out a big wail, and later really have a great belly laugh. What will it take to finally allow this emotional release?

Separation is about pulling away from painful memories of not being understood, feeling shame, being lonely, of never feeling my family or few friends from childhood ever truly knew how special I was.

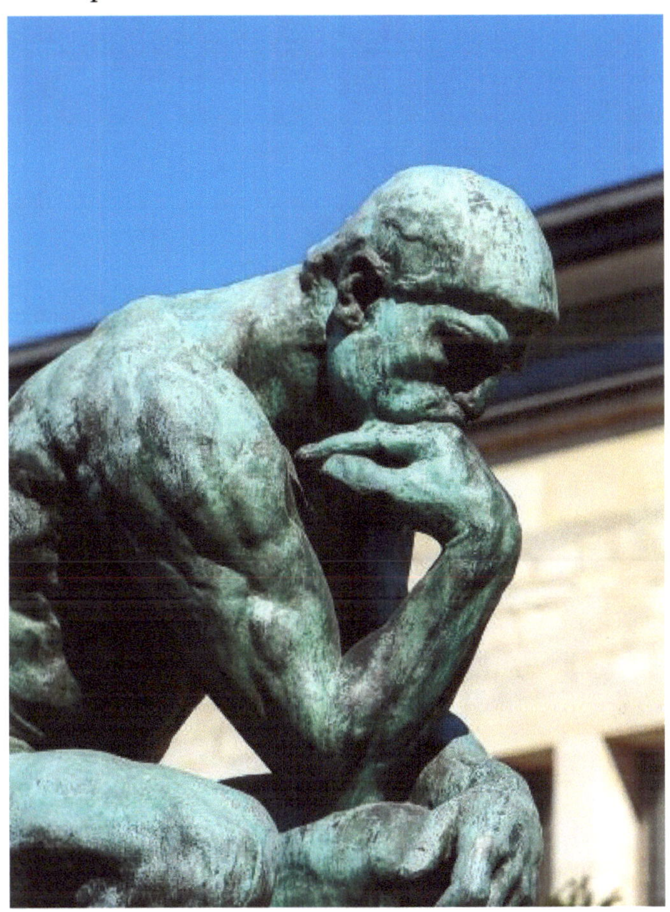

© Wjarek / Adobe Stock

This is the separation part of my personal "locked" safe. Through the emotional work which I did during my multiple stays at the Dead Sea, I can now release this feeling which is no longer relevant. I am now moving on to separate from the past pain. I made a declaration to be understood by others now and in the future. I told myself, I am not lonely anymore, I am special and don't need others to see this...even if I prefer they do. Through these types of positive declarations, I can release emotions which have kept my skin toxic and irritated.

There's lost love, unfinished conversations, missed opportunities, unfortunate handling of situations that caused others pain or embarrassment. These circumstances are not part of me now, nor were they intentional. Perceptions I once had including sadness, regrets, and feelings others may have had toward me mattered way too much and caused me to feel shame. This shadow engulfed me and subsequently, through time and layers of embarrassment, affected my overall health and erupted my skin. At the Dead Sea, I experienced a dissolving of this feeling about myself at the same exact moment I shed my skin for a fresh layer of baby skin. I was cleansed by the sea and special sunrays.

After experiencing separation, I began parts two and three—letting go and forgiving.

What of those people I've hurt? Was it real or imagined? If I did not mean to do it, did this make the hurt any less bearable? No, of course not! What of those who hurt me? Should either party go on punishing the other? I'm currently 63, when does the suffering finally end? Can we ever stop punishing ourselves?

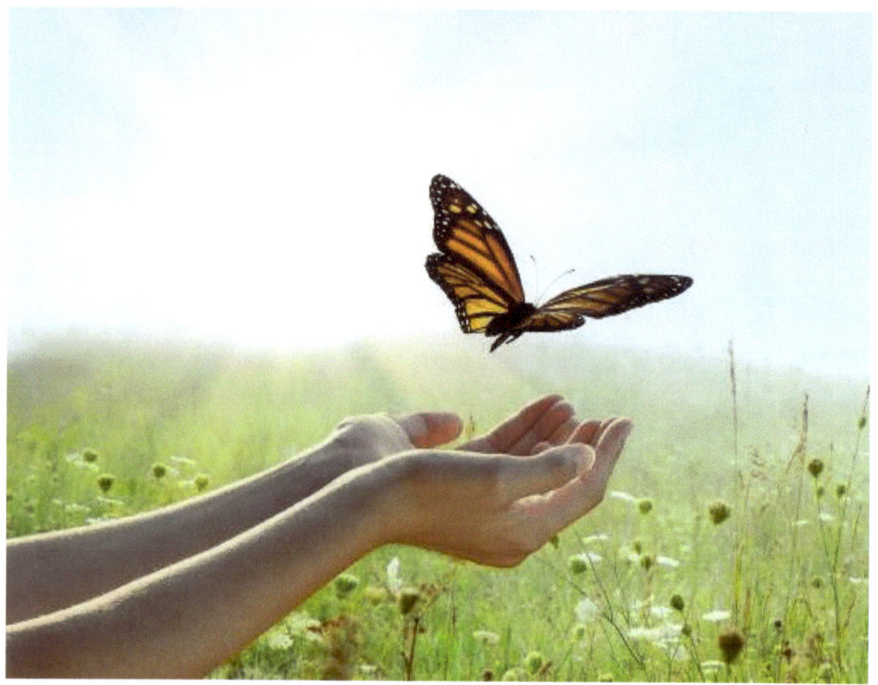

© *Lisa / Adobe Stock*

How much more life can be passed by without expressing the love and admiration for those I've met? Each person has blessed me, just by being there to teach me vital lessons. Each of these souls, dead or alive, gave me more compassion, empowering me with strength to go on. It's all part of the continuum of life. These lessons learned are never bad if we use them to help ourselves grow and teach others how to heal.

**August 14, 2007** – Today I'm feeling great! Skin was really smoothing out. I started to get to know people who came to this clinic and seaside resort every summer. It seemed there was a "club" of regular attendees tanning their flaky red psoriasis away in the nude on the rooftop. I now was a member of this club.

Some came for yearly tune-ups, but for the most part, were very much improved, if not completely in remission. The general attitude, especially among Israelis, was that each person is unique, and you must listen to your skin. At one time or another, all of them were patients of the clinic.

One Israeli told me he now self-monitors his skin since he's come there many years. His key was to relax and give up clock watching, TV, computer and cell phone communications, etc. You must give in to this process, really take time to be inside yourself and let go. This was my struggle. How to accomplish this on vacation should not be so difficult...I'm free now to become a new me. I pondered, *What's holding me back?*

**August 15, 2007** – Midway on my healing journey, I had about 13 more days at the Dead Sea. So, I took a break, calling it a mental and physical health day off. A few of my friends were noticing me getting a little red, not quite burnt, so I went to the clinic. They recommended my staying in the shade all day, applying a special cream after bathing in the indoor Dead Sea spa. I stayed there, read, relaxed, bathed and slept most of the day. It was just the tonic I needed as my body was beginning to tire from so much sun.

There absolutely is a balance at the Dead Sea and each person needs to find the appropriate level of sun/sea they can tolerate. This is what the doctor is for and how the clinic keeps you safely balanced and in check.

If you get sunburnt or worse, sunstroke, you risk losing three to four valuable days of expensive treatment. Gratefully, I just relaxed more during that one day. I'm happy about this decision not to push myself. There were still two weeks to finish my skin clearing.

**August 16, 2007** – I returned to the sun and sea today without feeling any burning. My skin took on a deeper tan, but at the same time, some of the Israeli patients noticed that new skin was forming and coming out from under where the pink/red areas previously were. A very nice Israeli man named Yaakov gave me some powerful words of encouragement. He told me that when I returned to the States, my wife would see me as a new man with the "skin of a baby!" This made me so happy inside to think that all of these years of struggle with this illness may be almost over. Wow!

Meanwhile, I continued to read more healing and spiritual books.

The next afternoon I would go on a weekend Sabbath retreat. I was invited to a town called Arad, high above the Dead Sea. A wonderful family nearby offered to have me for Friday night Sabbath dinner and the next day of prayer services. I was sincerely missing this feeling of being with my family and having a nice home cooked meal. It turned out to be a wonderful getaway and also allowed my skin another day to mature and grow anew.

**August 19, 2007** – It was a day of progressive reading and more nurturing sunrays. I began to realize that a huge part of my psoriasis came from negative feelings as well as environmental and possibly toxic relationships. Could that be possible? Either way you look at it, they are all poisonous to the system if they induce stress. To rid myself of this illness, I must purge these toxins and any bad feelings by a combination of positive nutrition and lots of liquids (detox teas and purified water) as well as the cultivation of "my happy thoughts" just like in the fairytale, *Peter Pan.*

My happy thoughts have always been my wife and children, but in the world outside of this my thoughts must become love (for thyself first...then others), compassion and unconditional generosity.

We've already discussed the power of forgiveness, patience and tolerance as a part of this powerful faith and mind training. The purpose behind this continuous work is to become the best possible me and to arrive at the place in my life where guilt about the past and fear about the future don't exist anymore.

**August 20, 2007** – This became my breakthrough day for my skin and emotions. I realized how much of me had been living a life of tentativeness and underlying fears. That morning something conjured up old fears inside me. On this day, I fought an old demon and slew it! It felt terrific, as if I had conquered something really big.

Among our rooftop gang of "psoriasis healing guys" my new friend Yaakov soon became a leader for all to look up to. As we had been suntanning regularly on the rooftop of the hotel, we decided to go on a fun field trip together.

Yaakov was very charming and funny. He reminded me of Yoda, the little fuzzy Jedi master in *Star Wars* because he was full of quick one-line philosophies. He seemed well-read and spoke eloquent English. Most importantly, I found in him a kind, understanding friend. Again, here's a recurring need for me to find a strong mentor/guide.

He invited me to see a nearby oasis in the hills near our hotel. Yaakov said, "We, our 'psoriasis gang' will meet at 11:13 in the lobby, so come with a towel, a water bottle and a camera, if you like." I said, "Who's driving us there?" like a typical American tourist. He replied, "No one, we're hiking. It's only 20 minutes or so!" My knee-jerk reaction about walking under the noonday sun around the Dead Sea was that it was totally forbidden by my doctor.

Also, I recalled another scary memory from my youth. It was in the hot Arizona desert over 40 years ago. At a sleep-away camp in Tucson, a group of students hiking in the desert, ran out of water and became dangerously dehydrated. Needing to be rescued fast, my roommate, a courageous 15-year old Israeli named Yisroel, ran for help. He alone had the stamina to achieve this miracle, coming from Israel's desert region. Therefore, I imagined us also getting dehydrated and running out of water in these desert hills.

All of my past fears about this misadventure from my teens resurfaced. Wow. I thought, *my skin is actually a memory organ where stress and fears can resurface and stick.*

Then, Yaakov simply said, "It's okay, you don't have to come, it's not the military." That did it! Now I felt challenged. Quickly I said I was coming. This was the best decision I'd made in all my time at the Dead Sea. I sensed I would feel wonderful on this group hike with Yaakov as our guide.

While I waited in the lobby for everyone to show up, promptly at 11:13, I saw the clock go beyond 11:25. I asked myself *why?* I began to feel worried and even somewhat abandoned. My thoughts ran wild, *did they leave without me?*

It was as if he was playing a joke and the whole group might not even come. I now see I feared something else which was very old. It was how my mother repeatedly told me her father died of a heart attack when she was only six. Her mother, uncles and aunts insisted she be brought over to say goodbye to her dead father. How strange! She was only a little girl.

Yet, in my 50s, I had internalized and empathized with her imprinted memory. Every time anyone died or even left town...she reenacted this drama, goodbye always felt like rejection. I too was feeling as if Yaakov had abandoned me, just like my mother felt her father had. Maybe it was because I really liked Yaakov, looked up to him and envisioned him as a father figure.

It started to make sense that I was worried about Yaakov coming to the hotel lobby. I called his room, he laughed and said, "I told you I'd be there at 11:30, were you worried I wouldn't come?" I was ashamed to say yes but instead told him, "No I had misunderstood the time."

Seriously, with his accent, I did hear it wrong. I had heard "eleven thirteen" and he actually said "thir-ty" with his Hebrew accent. It's reasonable to see how I could have been unclear. However, I'm sure it was G-d's way of testing my recurring fears of abandonment. And this replaying of old fears and facing them has helped me to further develop my ideas about what causes psoriasis.

And so, at precisely 11:30 am, we embarked up the mountain trail with our fearless and proud Yaakov leading the group. Soon we were marching into a beautiful valley of green bushes, flowing brooks, all between ancient sculpted rocks. Climbing higher, we discovered waterfalls and small joyful swimming pools in which we swam to cool off during the midday heat. We had so much fun...without a care in the world. My old fears of being dehydrated in the noonday sun evaporated miraculously.

That evening, my 19-year old daughter could hardly believe her ears as I called and told her how daddy actually climbed a mountain trail like a young billy goat. I felt renewed and invigorated because I had triumphantly overcome an old fear of hiking in the desert. At the same time, I released that horrible memory of death, abandonment and rejection about which my mother repeatedly anguished her whole life.

**August 21, 2007, philosophy of Yaakov** – I began to admire Yaakov more and wanted to know how he dealt with his own suffering in life. What was his answer? He had a simple approach toward psoriasis. "It's really nothing," he chuckled. "Just be positive and stop punishing yourself!" He confounded me again with his laughter as I was reading one of my intellectual guidebooks to healing. He said, "Stop thinking about it as an illness. We are special and unique, better than the average person because we are a 'brotherhood of zebras.' Our stripes are beautiful. We can share and communicate with each other freely! Just like stripped zebras in Africa, we stand out amidst ordinary horses."

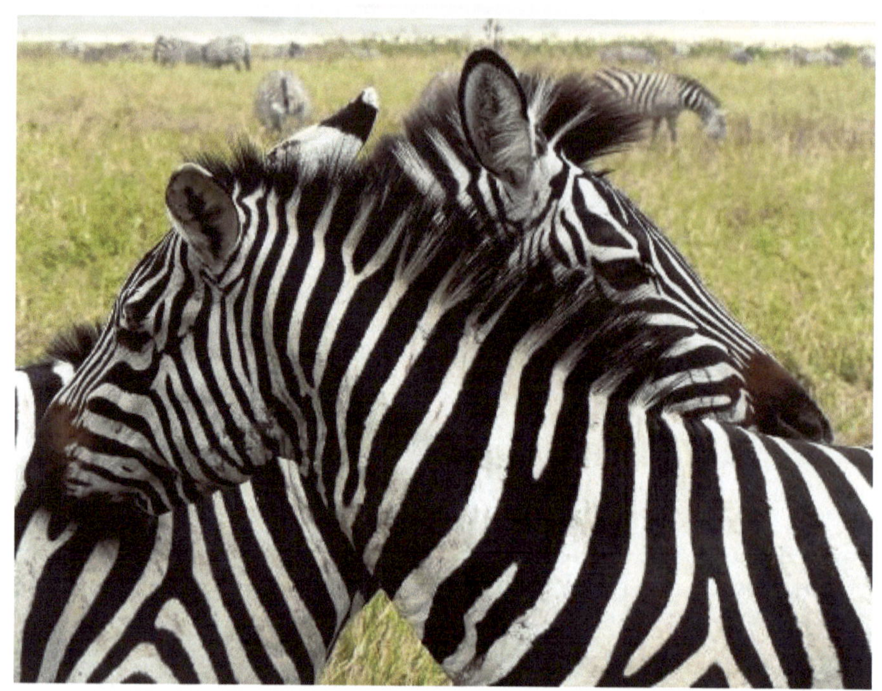

*© Steve / Adobe Stock*

This is the kind of amazing free philosophy I received upon the rooftop as we tanned in the nude. Part of me wanted to say, *he's right, get off of it and just enjoy the rest of your life day-by-day.* He simplified things...yet, there was more work involved for me, and I think for other dysfunctional people. I believed in my heart that Yaakov was extremely unique from all others I'd met at the Dead Sea. He didn't need group feedback, approval or love. Somehow, he engendered the spirit of someone who'd psychologically overcome his illness. It was not an obstacle to him anymore. He already arrived at a state of confidence and self-love. It was amazing for me to witness.

**August 22-23, 2007, Icarus crashed** – Yesterday morning, my doctor told me I was lesion free. Finally, after 23 years with both arthritis and chronic psoriasis, I could go home healthy, after just 19 days of treatment. Well, this got to my head and I stayed in the sun a little too long. This time I found myself just like the young Greek mythological Icarus who flew too close to the sun. It's been told that his ego allowed him to soar as his wax wings melted, and so he plummeted to Earth. I also was having too much fun and sun!

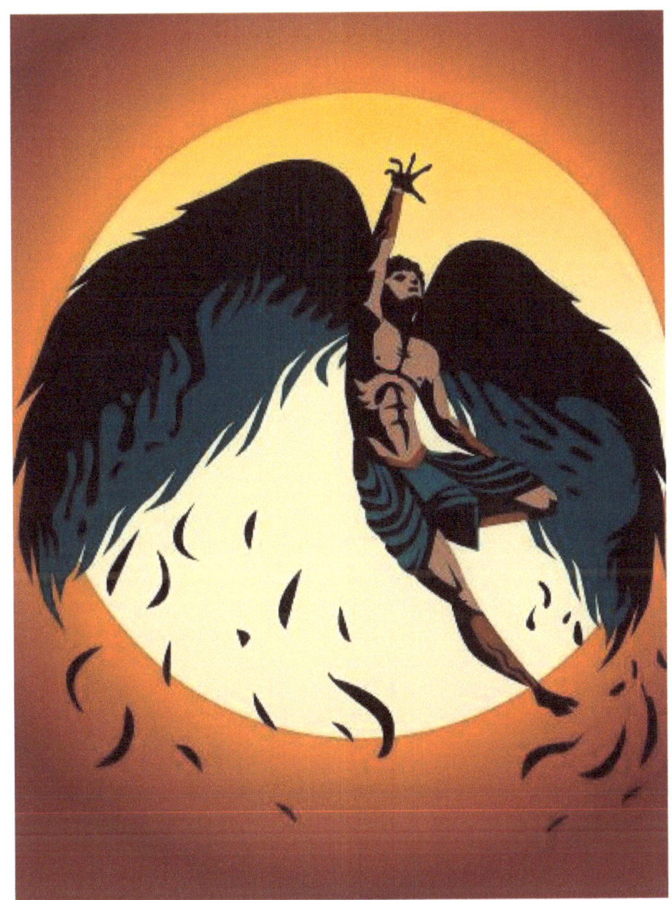



I felt nauseous, had the shivers and woke up not feeling right. As I went to the indoor Dead Sea waters in the morning, I noticed my skin having pimple eruptions and went back to the clinic to ask them what to do. They gave me a zinc cream formula for the skin eruptions and told me to read, rest and relax. No sun for a day or so.

My doctor told me my immune system was lower from all of the sea and sun treatment, which would be fine, not to worry. But then, after we finished on the rooftop the previous night, two of my friends encouraged me to go and celebrate my clear skin with a bit of Scotch whiskey. I didn't want to partake but felt if I refused this would be inhospitable. After one sip of this strong alcohol, I knew I would be completely ill. At dinner, I knew it in my gut I would not be able to stomach any food. So, I went upstairs at about 8:30 exhausted and crashed on my bed until 7 am the next day.

The lesson in all of this is never, ever overdo it at the Dead Sea. Be careful, especially when you are making progress, and I was reminded after this bad experience—never drink alcohol during the treatments. Obviously, it had a very bad effect.

**August 24, 25, 26, 2007** – This was my final Sabbath at the Dead Sea clinic and it was spent largely socializing and saying goodbye to the wonderful friends I met during my stay. We had all affected each other positively in our special healing process with lots of laughter, shooting pool, and dipping together in the warm mineral sea at night. Together we observed the evening splendor of the moon and stars on the glimmering waters which reflected red mountains.

The next day at 5 am, I was finally fortunate to make the spectacular morning climb to the ancient fortress of Masada with three other friends.

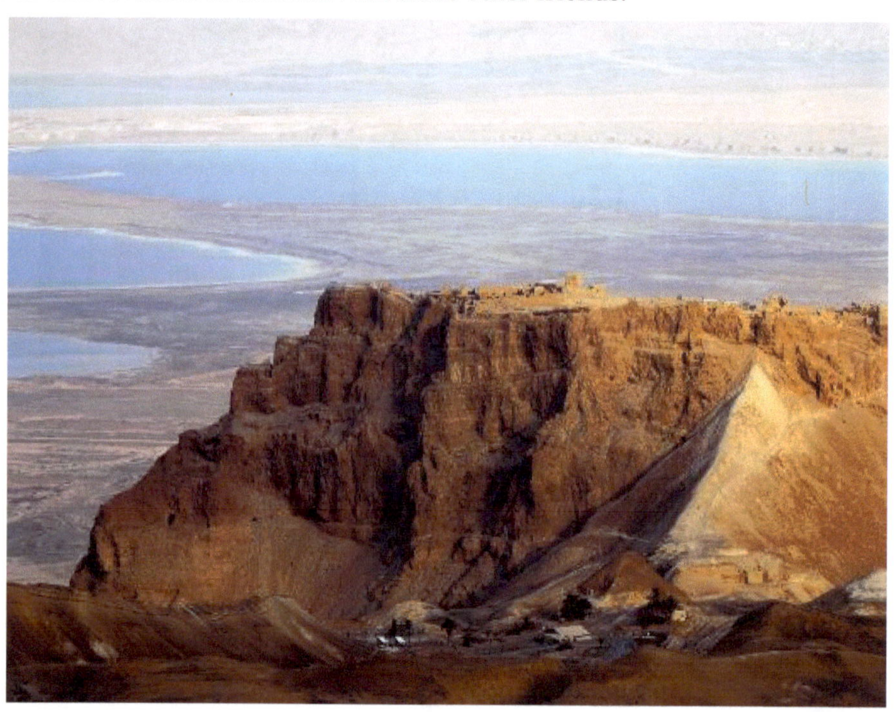

*© Ravan Even / Adobe Stock*

Earlier, I spoke about how history says there is evidence that this mountaintop was the final holdout (equal to the Alamo in the American Western days) by a band of rebel Jews who fought and died (some say by suicide to avoid capture) against a multitude legion of Roman conquerors. It took place shortly after the fall of the Second Temple. It was a breathtaking and inspirational journey to the top at dawn. As we climbed and watched the sunrise, we appreciated the grandeur and history of this landmark palace of the Jewish Nation.

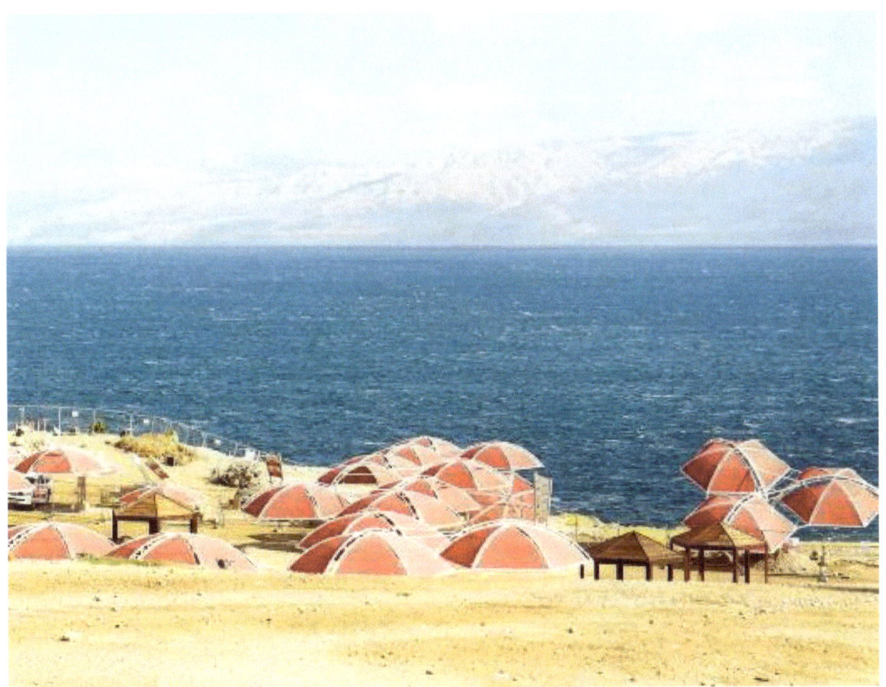

Later the same day, I had a final morning soak in the Dead Sea. I then took a day trip to Jerusalem and for the second time in my life I was able to pray at the *Kotel* (the Western Wall of the Second Temple) which is the only part still standing. The rest was destroyed by those same horrible Romans who pillaged Masada.

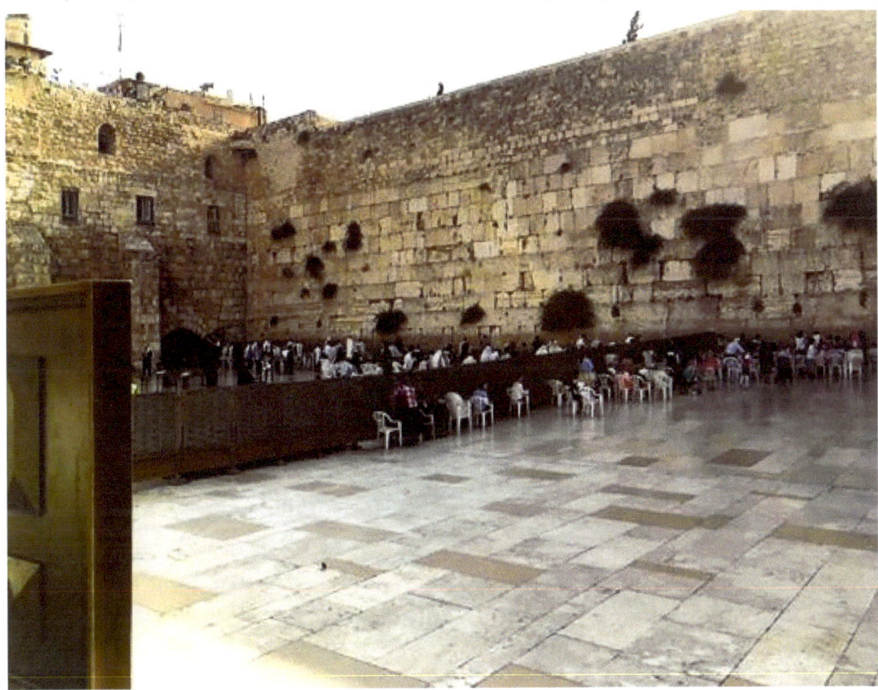

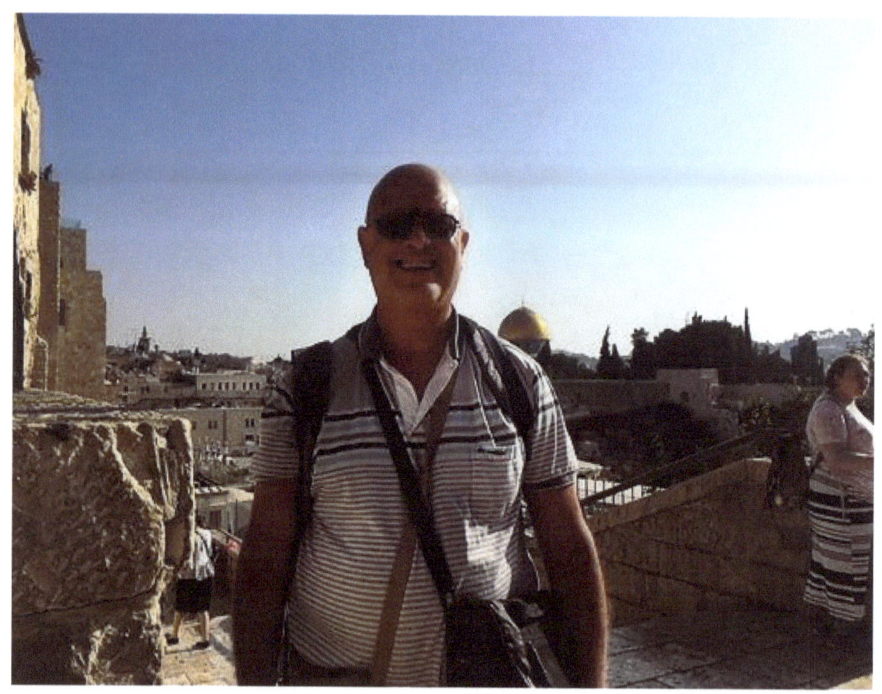

What does all of this have to do with treatment of my psoriasis? Well, just taking time off to heal between intense sessions in the sun turned out to be an important part of my recovery. As you've seen in the video clip, I reached my goal of total clearing by my 18-20th day. The rest of my time at the Dead Sea was dedicated to getting more benefits, but not to stress out about any further hard work on my healing. I could now just have fun. The Dead Sea is a recreational spot for many without skin issues, and Israel has so much more to offer any visitor who has extra days to see its sites and meet its wonderful people.

**August 27, 2007** – On the day before my departure, my doctor told me I was one of his best cases because I worked hard and carefully followed the process. In a recent email, he reiterated that I was an icon of success. I asked very good questions, he added, and said someday I would help a lot of people with my positive attitude.

**August 29, 2007, my last hours at the Dead Sea clinic** – As I prepared to depart on my journey back to the USA, I thought of the hard work I had accomplished. The sea was warm and extraordinarily nurturing. I still revel in this miraculous sun which beat the "heck" out of my skin...to the point where I was finally free of psoriatic lesions.

I knew then that the continuing remission process would be up to me. I planned to maintain my health by lowering stress levels, improving my positive attitude and enjoying a balanced nutritional diet. I knew I would have to cope with difficult situations better than ever, increase my level of spiritual awareness and remain emotionally stable. As they say, "If it's going to be, it's up to me!"

I returned home focused not to fall into the old habit patterns which I recently had broken out of, such as my old reaction to daily stresses, confusion, getting overwhelmed and stuck in bad thinking. My new life had to be one of change and mindful health, with a keen awareness of what would be best for the "ex-psoriasis" patient. This is a lifestyle lesson, and only I could make this commitment. I believe that in these days and weeks away from the USA, I came in touch with my own issues. My union with kindhearted and supportive psoriasis brothers and sisters at the Dead Sea fueled the desire to succeed and create this book. The entire experience has enabled me to share this document to encourage sane living for all of us to draw upon.

Saying goodbye to all of my new friends in 2007 was very difficult, however, saying farewell to my illness of over 23 years was not. I realized that often through struggle and much adversity comes success. I was blessed to have had this condition for it has made me sensitive to myself as well as to others. It also made me discover my love for Israel, the Land and its people. It became my healing and happy zone...I will never give up this love and dream to stay close to my new country.

I can declare how *I now do love myself* as never before and am able to give back and love all of my fellows equally, without judgment. This process is a divine and heaven-sent gift. I believe we can all achieve this state of mind.

**August 30, 2007, departing the airport for home** – My last evening in Israel, before returning to my wife and children in the USA, I kept another promise to myself. I went from the Dead Sea hotel to a religious village outside of Tel Aviv, and stayed with a close rabbi friend, Fish Jacobs and his wonderful family. The next day he introduced me to a world-famous spiritual guru and mathematical genius who had dedicated his life to understanding spiritual geometry and Kabbalistic healing. His name is Rabbi Ginsberg – see more at http://www.inner.org/rav and his soft-spoken approach to teaching left me with yet another great way to be attentive to others along the way. This experience was a wonderful way for me to end my first journey to the Dead Sea with inspiration and solace. I suggest reading his wonderful book, *Kabbalah of Body, Mind & Soul.*

## EPILOGUE

Two months after returning from this experience my memories were still quite vivid. I still felt the dry hot soothing Dead Sea and the intense healing rays of the sun. I had finally finished reading *Timeless Healing, The Power and Biology of Belief* by Herbert Benson, M.D. which was the last book on the recommended list from Dr. Botwick. It helped me to see how my healing journey continues. Clearly, I will always be involved with my inner work of improvement and change.

Even though some of the spots might return, I knew I could always return to Israel to clear completely, but more importantly, I had the mind/body/spiritual motivation to work on many areas of my life to live healthily and with meaning.

As Dr. Benson discussed (p. 275), choose not to think so anxiously. In the worse case scenario, always slow down and ask, what can happen, why am I allowing myself to worry, breathe in and out...relax and try redirecting this negative flow into a good direction. Utilize music, singing, art, cooking, exercise, and fun. His method of listening to ourselves, stopping to breathe and releasing all tension can both diminish, and eventually, break our habit of doom and gloom to help reprogram us into a positive healing lifestyle.

Are you ready to make a similar journey to healing? I hope you will go to the Dead Sea clinic to clear your skin.

## Spiritual work that can help

This is an open door to your soul. Many roads may be taken. Find a rabbi, preacher, guru or mentor with whom you can discuss spiritual cleansing and healing. This is your path. I am working on using music I love to hear and dance to, Qigong exercise/release, and Kabbalah teaching to help me in my continued healing. Choose the path that is right for you.

## Psychological antidotes to psoriasis

I developed my Un-Psoriasis Theory to find ways to reverse my condition. Late one night, I arrived at this idea because we all have our polarities, going through emotional up's and down's, in's and out's, so I surmised that psoriasis must also have its opposite side. I therefore coined the phrase Un-Psoriasis Theory. Every person with psoriasis has known triggers. If you ask them they can usually identify when psoriasis began and what preceded it.

I began to hypothesize with my psoriasis friends that we all had some unresolved issues in our youth which we believed may have contributed to our condition. Without a great deal of research, I asked them to each reflect on the idea of challenges they have faced and also any blessings they were willing to speak about.

The idea behind this is that we are a part of a world with many opposites, such as up/down, light/dark, inside/outside. We live in a world of yins and yangs.

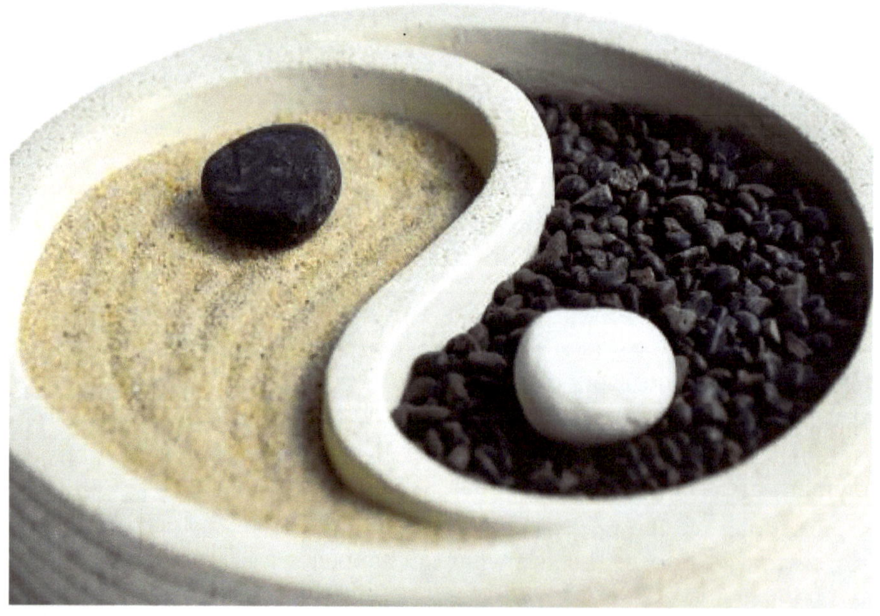

© *Pegasosart / Adobe Stock*

I concluded from my friends' feedback that if psoriasis can exist, it must have an underlying cause and an opposite such as "un-psoriasis." If we can restore or repair what may have been a challenge for us individually, then it might be possible for us to again harvest the blessing of our youthful good health. None of the people I'd interviewed had been born with psoriasis. It happened suddenly after some unique trauma.

In studying all of the responses, I developed a list of opposite traits. Originally, I wrote them on a deck of 52 playing cards. I placed one concept on the face of a card, with its opposite on the reverse side. This deck of cards enabled me to review how I was feeling daily by flipping them over and being honest with myself about these opposite emotions.

Anytime you feel that you lean toward having elements or even emotional reactions in the *Negative emotions* left column, try to work on and grow yourself toward the *Positive emotions* right column using meditation, prayer and self-love attitudes.

| Negative emotions | Positive emotions |
| --- | --- |
| Paralyzed, stuck, helpless | Enthusiastic, excited, beaming! |
| Irresponsible, guiltless | Responsible and Accountable |
| Feverous, exhausted, overworked | Alive, vigorous, energetic |
| Un-friendly | Friendly |
| Strange, disturbed | Human, real, calming |
| Fearful, worried, anxious | Courageous, brave |
| Intolerant, un-accepting | Understanding |
| Excluded, non-essential | Indispensable, included |
| Mean, annoyed | Compassionate |
| Greedy, selfish | Generous |
| Taking others for granted | Devoted and caring |
| Intolerant, un-accepting | Empathetic |
| Rude | Considerate |
| Violent | Gentle |
| Shut-down | Open |
| Dissatisfied, frustrated | Content, satisfied |
| Two-faced, absurd | Sincere |
| Misunderstood, feeling stupid & ridiculous | Accepted, understood, appreciated |
| Cruel, disturbed | Kind |
| Rejected, hopeless, miserable | Desired |
| Angry, bitter | Delighted |
| Distant, cold | Warm |
| Crumbled, made a fool of | Chivalrous |
| Mistreated, demoralized | Respected |
| Disgusted, turned-off | Enchanted, blissful |
| Hurt, contemptible | Loved, admired |
| Insecure, threatened, vulnerable, resentful | Secure |

| Negative emotions | Positive emotions |
| --- | --- |
| Torn apart, diminished | Happy, joyous, fulfilled |
| Betrayal, abandonment, jealousy, fear of loss, fear of failure | Loyalty, trust, adoration, commitment to another |
| Stressed-out, shaken, shy, shattered | Confident |
| Uncertain, indecisive | Determined, decided |
| Unappreciated, ungrateful | Thankful for all of our blessings |
| Restless, hostile, furious, agressive | Peaceful |
| Impatient, irritated, anxious, tormented | Patient |
| Confused, lost, unfocused | Centered |
| Distracted | Alert |
| Puny, powerless, weak | Powerful, solid, sturdy |
| Disunited, independent, sole | Unified |
| Deprived, belittled | Fortunate |
| General, ordinary | Special |
| Dark, lacking charm | Radiating |
| Impassionate, cold | Passionate |
| Commonplace, familiar | Fantastic |
| Affected | Unaffected, firm, strong |
| Bored | Fascinated |
| Threatened, intimidated, useless | Competent |
| Despised, detested, unimportant | Important, esteemed |
| Depressed, miserable, sorry, unhappy | Thrilled |
| Overburdened, overwhelmed | Comfortable |
| Looked-down upon | Envied, looked-up to with pride |
| Dishonest | Frank, honest, sincere |

## Health food suggestions for autoimmune conditions

On my own, I researched and discovered it's good to eat oily fish like trout, mackerel, salmon, sardines, and herring. Foods like poultry, eggs, and lamb should be eaten infrequently, and red meat very sparingly. All nuts are okay (except peanuts). Eat fruits and liquids before a meal, never during or for one full hour after. I have heard several times from nutritionists that there is something about having sweets, such as fruit right before a meal to aid digestion.

Here are the no's, sorry...ouch! We are not supposed to have these items since they can really aggravate our digestive system and skin even more. The benefit is you will look great and lose weight as well. I know, most of us love pizza, pasta, pork, etc. What's with this? Well, they are just not good for us.

Also, many people have reactions to milk, cheese, yogurt, tofu or soy milk, cereals or grains (gluten). No sugar or alcohol. No beans like navy, kidney, black, red, refried (skip all Mexican food), no Indian chickpeas, or split pea soup.

Our general goal is to restore all liver and digestive functions.

I recommend reading Dr. Steven Gundry's *Plant Paradox* book – located at www.gundrymd.com/plant-paradox-shopping-list/ for those interested in an even more strict program which some believe will enable chronic psoriasis and other autoimmune conditions to go into remission.

## Healing psoriasis from the inside

While there will never be something that works for everyone, I believe people can strive for better health by tweaking this program individually. After all, we are all "chromoso-matically" different, even though we have many biological similarities.

What I see through all of this self-analysis is that we are incomplete beings. Just as the world is evolving and needs constant looking after (as in a concept called *Tikkun Olam* in Jewish philosophy), we also need repairs. It's as if we are all being "recalled" by the Almighty manufacturer for upgrades and new parts.

Let us look at our current state as something we entered at a specific moment in time. I wondered, *how can we return to the period prior to the illness?* What was our state of mind and attitude like back then, before we got psoriasis symptoms? Can we pray for guidance on reviving this feeling? Is there a way to return, "through the eye of the needle" metaphorically, to once again become healthy and youthful? Many alternative practitioners have real case histories of such remarkable restorative healings. How about you and me too?

Dr. Benson asserts in *Timeless Healing* that we are able to recall a time of wellness. He believes (p. 44) faith or a serious longing can create a healing result. It actually helps our bodies recall the messages and the instructions associated with that which we long for. In other words, our subconscious mind will follow these instructions out of pure faith, creating the results. This strong faith factor must be embedded in our wellness.

Suggested future healing activities are to sing happy songs from your innocent childhood, enjoy music and movies from great times before illness occurred, and visualize a phrase or mantra which will aid you in returning to a state of calm should stress return.

Herein exists the total rub...if people are convinced by doctors and the claim of inevitable recurrence of some lesions, then the panic of the old wounds which caused this illness may also return. This belief will circularly aggravate the condition even more. We need to enter a Zen mode of response to stress and fears. Instead of a fight or flight reaction, it must become a calm and meditative transition into the Remembered Wellness process which is in the *Timeless Healing* book. This process must bring us into the zone of the original womb, of being taken care of and loved. But now, as an adult we must transform this into self-love nurturing, as it's the only solution to wellness. It's an inside game.

Ultimately, this must be achieved alone, even if we love the group of people or family members who may wish to help us get there. That support must be temporary. No one can do the major job of staying the lonely course of becoming "one" and strong again...even the caring club of other wounded people becomes a perpetrator of recurring psoriasis. As a result of not wanting to lose the new support of friendships we have cherished, we might cling to this "newfound psoriasis family" that understands us better than our own family ever could. In this way, we may take the chance of hurting ourselves even more by returning to a state of illness, not wishing to leave these close companions.

The solution may be to create a separate "graduates club" perhaps not located at the Dead Sea. It could be an island resort in a Mediterranean region, a relaxing hot spring, or even a meditation retreat. We might meet in the winter months, not to brag, but to rejoice about our remarkable success in beating the very slim odds of a permanent remission, which the medical world declares unlikely.

This must be our ardent goal even if some of us return to the Dead Sea for intermittent tune-ups. It's okay to fix the small recurring minor lesions occasionally in the future. It may, in fact, take two to three seasons or even years in a row to break old habits and reset our autoimmune system on the right track with proper diet, digestion, elimination, attitude and commitment level. We must believe this is worth it...that we are worth it, no matter the cost!

It is known that talk therapy is highly effective in prolonging remission among psoriasis patients. We must also stay clean of toxic foods and substances. There are also toxic ideas and words...even toxic relationships which keep us from healing and advancing. Accepting this last statement may be the toughest pill to swallow in our work toward ultimate healing. What if there really are people in our lives who are bad for our health? Do we stay close to them? Should we and can we distance ourselves from them? Is it worth living more independently—alive—than living together, one or both getting even more sick?

It's important not to harbor resentments. We can only stay healthy if we control our mind, body and spirit from impurity. We must detoxify on every level. It's our decision. Make it with me.


## CONCLUSION

After returning to the USA from my visit in 2017, I made a resolution to work exclusively on nutrition, exercise and my stress level. Here are the results of this approach which I call "to thine own self be true" to add Shakespeare's quote to the mix.

Many years ago, I read about the Leaky Gut Syndrome in several works, *The Yeast Connection* by Dr. William Crook, written in 1986 and *One Cause, Many Ailments: The Leaky Gut Syndrome* by Dr. John Pagano, written in 2008. Both books opened my mind to how the gut is a major source of stress and illness.

Dr. Gundry agrees with easing the congestion in the gut to allow for optimal digestion and elimination. The Black Hebrews of Dimona also believe in this technique of healing using their vegan diets with periodic fasting. Many groups and doctors practice this path of lowering stress and making our insides work properly in order to allow "inside-out" detox and cleansing. Hippocrates stated, "All disease begins in the gut."

Another article, *How to Heal Leaky Gut Syndrome in 4 Simple, Tasty Steps*, published April 2017 at blog.kettleandfire.com/how-to-heal-leaky-gut-syndrome, states that many studies find gut issues are the root of autoimmune and other diseases, including chronic fatigue, bloating, joint pains, and skin problems. People with this root cause may crave sugar, carbs and become sensitive to certain foods which exacerbate their condition.

Remember the saying *you are what you eat*. While some people are affected more by certain foods, others can eat anything and not get a reaction. Many are lactose or gluten intolerant as is seen in the thousands of new products in the supermarkets in the USA and elsewhere. We also see major growth in distribution of organically grown and natural products at health food stores and online for every type of ailment.

I believe my gut was compromised along with other organs of digestion and elimination, leaving my skin as the only detox and purging outlet. It truly is the major organ/system of perspiration and detoxification and it comes to the rescue when all other organs fail. Remember, the skin completely surrounds us. If it could not breathe in or exhale to eliminate, we'd simply die, just like James Bond's girlfriend did in the movie *Goldfinger* when the bad guys covered her entirely with gold paint.

My gut has been leaking particles into my bloodstream which were meant to go into my digestive track. When these random particles go into our blood it sets off immune system alarms screaming that foreign invaders have arrived. It's like an alien attack, and we try to combat it while our immune system's response is inflammation. Potential chronic versions can start with psoriasis or arthritis (non-life threatening ordinarily). However, they potentially promote 50% greater chance of high blood pressure (also stress induced), heart disease, cancers, stroke, and diabetes. These are in scientific research and are referred to as "comorbidities." For specific information go to this worldwide psoriasis patient site at www.psoriasis.org/about-psoriasis/related-conditions.

I have experienced many of the leaky gut symptoms: food sensitivities, psoriasis, irritable bowel, stomach conditions, mood disorders and depression. By treating the gut and overcoming Leaky Gut Syndrome, many issues can be healed.

# BIBLIOGRAPHY


*The Art of Happiness* by the Dalai Lama, 2009 – a Nobel Prize winner and spiritual leader of Tibet is a sought-after speaker and statesman. He's often peaceful and smiling, continually bringing this joy to all he meets, so everyone else around him feels like smiling.

*Spontaneous Healing* by Dr. Andrew Weil, 1995 – Dr. Weil teaches that our bodies can indeed spontaneously heal and it's a fact of biology—we are each born with this natural healing system.

*When All You've Ever Wanted Isn't Enough* by Rabbi Harold Kushner, 1986 – He writes this with compassion and wisdom similar to his bestseller *When Bad Things Happen to Good People*, Kushner's philosophies are universal and speak to us in a timeless way about seeking a meaningful life.

*Why People Don't Heal and How They Can* by Caroline Myss, Ph.D., 1994 – In this book, she creatively discusses how we need to believe in ourselves, and not talk ourselves into illness, before recovery can occur.

*Timeless Healing, The Power and Biology of Belief* by Herbert Benson, M.D., 1996 – In this life-changing book, Dr. Benson discusses and shows how affirming and more positive self-talk beliefs can change our current illness to more physical health.

*The Relaxation Response, a Simple Meditative Technique that will Unlock Your Hidden Assets*, by Herbert Benson, M.D., 1975 – A great methodology and health handbook to show techniques designed to reduce physiological stress and offer healing plus relaxation.

*Kabbalah of Body, Mind and Soul*, by Rabbi Yitzchak Ginsburg, 2014 – Rabbi Ginsburg, who I've met several times in Israel, is a wonderful calming teacher of this type of ancient healing Kabbalah. He offers us a way to maintain overall health plus spiritual well-being.

*The Plant Paradox* by Dr. Steven Gundry, 2017 – He's at the forefront of scientific knowledge. *The Plant Paradox* is a must-read book for anyone interested in total detox and rejuvenation.

###

www.HealthRightIsrael.com about the Dead Sea, health practitioners and longevity.